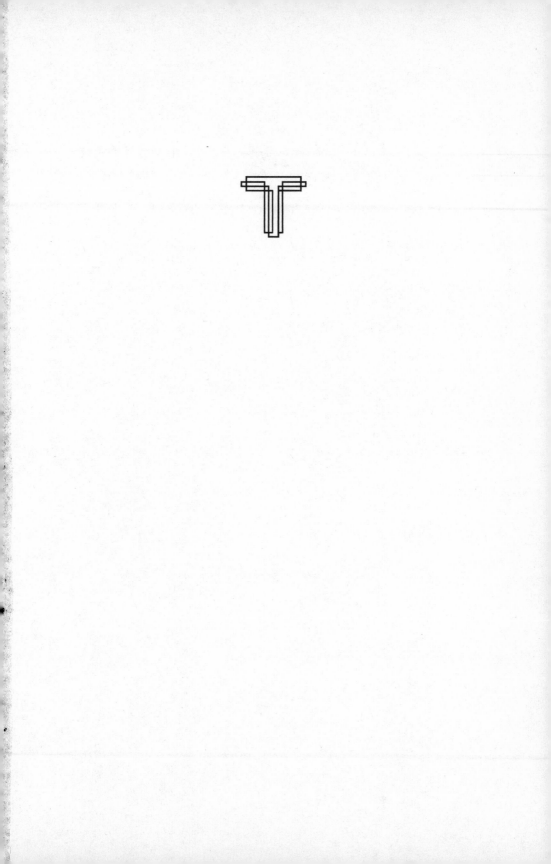

Cannabis for Chronic Pain

A PROVEN PRESCRIPTION FOR USING MARIJUANA TO **RELIEVE YOUR PAIN** AND **HEAL YOUR LIFE**

DR. RAV IVKER, DO, ABIHM

Cofounder and Former President,
American Board of Integrative Holistic Medicine

Former President, American Holistic Medical Association

TOUCHSTONE
New York   London   Toronto   Sydney   New Delhi

Touchstone
An Imprint of Simon & Schuster, Inc.
1230 Avenue of the Americas
New York, NY 10020

First Touchstone hardcover edition September 2017

TOUCHSTONE and colophon are registered trademarks of Simon & Schuster, Inc.

For information about special discounts for bulk purchases, please contact Simon & Schuster Special Sales at 1-866-506-1949 or business@simonandschuster.com.

The Simon & Schuster Speakers Bureau can bring authors to your live event. For more information or to book an event, contact the Simon & Schuster Speakers Bureau at 866-248-3049 or visit our website at www.simonspeakers.com.

Interior design by Kyle Kabel

Manufactured in the United States of America

10 9 8 7 6 5 4 3 2 1

Library of Congress Cataloging-in-Publication Data

Names: Ivker, Rav, author.
Title: Cannabis for chronic pain : a proven prescription for using marijuana to relieve your pain
    and heal your life / Dr. Rav Ivker, DO, ABIHM, co-founder and past president, American
    Board of Integrative Holistic Medicine, past president, American Holistic Medical Association.
Description: New York : Touchstone, 2017.
Identifiers: LCCN 2017025407| ISBN 9781501155888 (hardback) | ISBN 9781501155901
    (paperback) | ISBN 9781501155918 (ebook)
Subjects: LCSH: Marijuana—Therapeutic use. | Chronic pain—Treatment. | BISAC:
    MEDICAL / Holistic Medicine. | HEALTH & FITNESS / Pain Management. |
    MEDICAL / Drug Guides.
Classification: LCC RM666.C266 I95 2017 | DDC 615.3/23648—dc23
LC record available at https://lccn.loc.gov/2017025407

ISBN 978-1-5011-5588-8
ISBN 978-1-5011-5591-8 (ebook)

To my beloved Harriet,
who for the past fifty years has taught me most
of what I know about the art of loving

Contents

PART II
Self-Care 101: MMJ + Holistic Medicine = Long-Lasting Pain Relief

Introduction

Chronic Pain Is a Blessing Disguised as a Curse

Joy and Woe are woven fine, a clothing for the soul Divine. 'Neath every grief and pine, runs a joy with silken twine. Human beings are made for joy and woe, and when this we rightly know, through the world we safely go.

—William Blake, an English poet, painter,
and printmaker (1757–1827)

I awoke with the pain hitting me like a bolt of lightning, as if I were being electrocuted. I had never felt a pain like this.

The diagnosis was easy. The grotesque blistering rash resembling chicken pox protruding from purplish skin along the left side of my abdomen and around my left flank to my back was unmistakable.

During my forty-four years as a family doctor I'd seen many patients suffering with shingles and this was a classic textbook case. The pain I experienced on that early-spring morning in March 2015, which I rated a 7 on a scale of 1 to 10, would soon progress to an 8 or 9 as my *baseline* pain level—i.e., it never went below an 8. This baseline persisted for another two months.

By the end of that first week and lasting for another four weeks, I had 10s and even 10+s (off-the-chart pain)! I referred to the latter as *zingers*. Fortunately when they hit me they didn't last long. But my memory of them will remain vivid for the rest of my life. The zingers were flashes of excruciating pain, far beyond the baseline of an 8 and greater than a 10. I couldn't imagine a pain worse than this. They came out of nowhere, with absolutely no warning, and literally took my breath away, and I yelled as if I'd just been shot or stabbed in my belly. (I'm assuming the pain was similar since I've fortunately never had either experience. I've since been told by a patient who's endured both that the pain from shingles is actually worse than a gunshot.)

The zingers were totally incapacitating, and caused me to spontaneously curl up in a fetal position. This reflexive movement was my body's response—to try and protect itself, to stop the pain, and to prevent it from recurring, all at the same time.

In the flick of a switch that traumatized me, along with my T-10 spinal nerve, my former life disappeared. I had been transformed from a vibrantly healthy sixty-eight-year-old guy to a survivor cowering in fear of the jolts of pain. My mind's sole focus was riveted on relieving the agony. It was all-consuming.

To describe this as a humbling experience would be a gross understatement. For someone who had enjoyed a high degree of control through most of my adult life and had treated more than seventy thousand patients, I was now rendered completely powerless to affect what was happening to my body.

I found myself in a desperate situation, at the mercy of a vicious and relentless microscopic organism. I had absolutely no control of how my body reacted to the zingers. I was unable to stifle the screams and remain a silent sufferer. It felt like I was wearing an electrocuting belt strapped around my waist that was always turned on. And manning the control switch was a deranged, sadistic individual who took great pleasure in turning up the current to the max and zapping me whenever he chose.

My initial reaction to this horrific situation was to feel *anger* with myself. I was highly self-critical for having allowed myself to become so stressed that my immunity broke down to a point where I contracted the virus. "I know lots of stress management techniques. Why didn't I do them? And why didn't I get the shingles vaccine?" Such a simple preventive measure that I had failed to do. I also felt *anger* with God for allowing this to happen to me. "What did I do to deserve this?"

Shame was also included as part of my emotional pain; shame for being so physically weak that I had become vulnerable to the virus, when the primary focus of my personal and professional practice for the past thirty years had been optimal health—this was a long way from that state of well-being. I *grieved* and cried over the loss of my physical strength and vitality and a relatively happy life. They were gone, and I had no idea if I'd ever regain them. I had great *empathy* for the vast majority of my patients who were also suffering with chronic pain. But perhaps the emotion that I was least able to express was *fear*. I was afraid of the pain itself, and of the unknown. *How long would it last? Would I be able to relieve the pain enough to work, to play with my grandkids, and to enjoy my life again?*

Enduring chronic pain is like being tortured without any letup. *Chronic* means that to some extent *it's always there*, like a jammed switch that won't turn off. (Medically, it's defined as pain that persists beyond three months.) And if the pain level remains at a level 5 or higher, then you're presented with a formidable challenge in shifting your focus to anything else for more than a few minutes. The degree of difficulty in diverting attention away from the pain increases exponentially with each higher numeric rating. For me, pain beyond a 6 made it nearly impossible to function well. Other than the zingers that occurred throughout the first month, the pain persisted at a baseline level between 8 and 9 for more than two months and was never lower than a 5 baseline for the first six months. This was the case only when *not* using medical marijuana.

Never in my life had I experienced chronic pain or any pain even close to this intensity. As an athlete, I've certainly had my share of physical pain from broken bones, bruises, sprains, and strains, but nothing lasting longer than two or three weeks. Whatever the injury was, I usually noticed a slight pain reduction almost daily. The shingles pain, however, was constant and the improvement measured in weeks and months. During the first nine months, it would typically take from seven to nine weeks to reduce the baseline pain level by one degree. I learned during medical school that nerves can take an exceptionally long time to heal, but now I had been given an opportunity to personally experience just how slow that process can be.

The pharmaceutical options (primarily opioids) offered by my physician colleagues were not helpful. They were minimally effective at reducing the pain, but their side effects (drowsiness, nausea, constipation) only added to my misery and I was unable to function the way I needed to. I started to feel as if I'd been *cursed* as a result of having done something really awful and been given this virus as the worst possible punishment.

I cringe at the thought of what my life might have been like had I not decided to self-medicate with medical marijuana. Up to that point I'd seen more than six thousand patients suffering with chronic pain who were using medical marijuana as their primary analgesic. These patients were either seeking a state license to use it for the first time or, the majority of cases, renewing their license, which in Colorado is required annually. I heard repeatedly from my patients how much more effective (with no adverse side effects) cannabis was in relieving their pain than the narcotics they'd been prescribed. In some cases, they'd been taking a variety of opioids for many years and had developed dependence or, even worse, an addiction.

After first trying the conventional route during the first week, with disappointing results, I began using medical marijuana. It was miraculous! It consistently reduced the pain to tolerable levels of 3 to 4, allowing me to continue functioning at a reasonably high level. Although I always had pain, and zingers too during the first couple of months (they only occurred when I had *not* taken marijuana), I was successfully able to shift my focus, at least enough to have a life beyond shingles. I did not miss a day of work because of the shingles, and I was able to resume hiking.

By the second week of my struggle with shingles I was taking at least one medical marijuana product daily, and by week seven, my usage had increased to between five and six products per day! I was amazed with both its potency as an analgesic and my ability to function (the medical marijuana products most effective for pain are somewhat lower in THC—tetrahydrocannabinol, the psychoactive component— and higher in CBD—cannabidiol, the non-psychoactive analgesic and anti-inflammatory, than marijuana for recreational use). These are the two most common and most medicinal of the eighty or more cannabinoids in cannabis, and they work synergistically to relieve pain. What I personally experienced and researchers have also found is that the psychoactive effect of THC is somewhat mitigated by both CBD and severe pain—you don't get too high and are able to focus on your work.

Through a trial-and-error process and the valuable feedback I'd received from my patients and from medical marijuana dispensary owners and employees, my cannabis medicine chest came to include a vaporizer (inhaling without smoke), tinctures (liquid extract placed under the tongue), edibles, hash oils (concentrates dispensed in a syringe and ingested), transdermal patches, topicals, and tablets. Each method of administration had its own list of benefits and minimal liabilities.

Although marijuana was great for relieving the pain, I knew it wouldn't cure the problem. "But surely I'm not at risk for post-herpetic neuralgia," I thought—i.e., shingles pain persisting beyond three months. "That only happens to old and unhealthy people." Or so I thought. Wishful thinking!

Soon after exceeding the three-month mark, I began hearing stories of people who had suffered for a year or more. One woman told me her mother had had it for more than seven years and it never resolved. She died with it in her mid-eighties. My fear increased, and the more anxious I became the more the pain increased. At this point I was also becoming somewhat depressed.

I renewed my commitment to rid my body of this virulent virus. I tried a variety of alternative therapies recommended by several of my holistic medical colleagues, including David Perlmutter, MD, perhaps the world's most highly respected holistic neurologist (author of *Grain Brain* and his latest book, *Brain Maker*). Some of the recommendations I followed included: high-dose vitamin B12 injections, adenosine monophosphate (AMP) injections, high-dose IV vitamin C, acupuncture, Healing Touch, and neurofeedback, along with a host of supplements that I ingested daily, several of which were supposed to help with nerve healing. I suspect several of these treatment modalities helped in reducing baseline pain levels, but none of them made the dramatic difference I was hoping for.

There is no question that medical marijuana (*cannabis* is the botanical name for the herb) has been by far the most effective therapy for quickly relieving the pain. Beside the pain relief, while its effect lasted I actually felt quite good and enjoyed a nearly normal life. Rather than being completely overwhelmed by the pain, I found it possible with cannabis to shift my focus to working, exercising, playing with my grandchildren and my wife, and maintaining my responsibilities at home. I would describe it as having a decent life while living with chronic pain.

I had learned more than three decades earlier that through suffering with a chronic illness I was able to transform my life in ways I could never have imagined (or planned). Though in retrospect, chronic sinusitis seemed like a mild discomfort relative to the shingles, perhaps my most valuable lesson from it was that a health crisis can provide an excellent opportunity for turning lemons into lemonade. You may or may not cure the problem, but the lessons learned are vital to healing your life. I know it may seem counterintuitive, but chronic illness, dis-ease, and pain can potentially be a *blessing*, as long as you're open to that possibility.

It took me years to first recognize this truth. After an ENT specialist delivered his dismal prognosis in 1980, telling me "You'll have to live with it," I had spent nearly seven years developing a holistic medical treatment to cure chronic sinusitis. Although the dietary changes and supplements, indoor air modification, and daily nasal hygiene practices were helpful, it wasn't until I worked with a spiritual psychotherapist, Myron McClellan, for a full year (1986) that I was able to cure this so-called *incurable* condition. Chronic sinusitis is considered the world's most common respiratory condition, and conventional medicine has no consistently effective treatment for either curing or even significantly improving it.

What I learned through curing sinusitis via the body-mind-spirit connection was that *unconditional love is life's most powerful healer*, and *the perceived loss of love is our greatest health risk*. I realized that *anything is possible* and that pain and dis-ease are *messengers*. They get our attention like nothing else can. They're alerting us to largely unconscious emotional and spiritual pain resulting from the loss of love from ourselves (we tend to perceive it as the loss of love from others). This in turn weakens our immune system, which then becomes a significant contributor to our physical pain and dis-ease. In short, *love heals* and *the loss of love makes us sick and causes pain*. Fortunately we currently have a multitude of studies supporting *the science of connection—the healing power of love*.

Yet in spite of the fact that I'd been teaching these holistic healing principles to my patients and physician colleagues for the past three decades, they quickly faded from memory as soon as the shingles took over my life. My single-minded focus was to *get rid of the pain.*

However, once the baseline pain level subsided to below a 5, I was ready to address the *issues in the tissues.* In relieving the pain and at the same time heightening my awareness, medical marijuana helped me tremendously to better understand why I had contracted this virus at this particular time, and to recognize what I needed to learn from what had initially appeared to be a horrendous catastrophe. If it is your intention to address the emotional and spiritual causes of your dis-ease while learning invaluable lessons from your pain, cannabis can be a highly effective facilitator. "The Issues in the Tissues" section of each of the chapters in Part II will help you begin this process, and Part III will discuss it in more depth.

It's now nearly two years since I began this intensive life-changing course with shingles. I have to assume there's more for me to learn since I'm still enrolled and the pain is still present, although it rarely exceeds a 2. It's almost always there, but rather than it being all-consuming, I frequently have to shift my attention to even notice it.

Given this major improvement, it's been more challenging to stay fully engaged in the "shingles healing program," even though I'm already aware that the pain has served as a powerful catalyst for profoundly changing my life for the better. In spite of the precedent with sinusitis more than thirty years ago, it still amazes me that as I continue to heal, I'm feeling *blessed* by the shingles virus and its intense physical pain. It has brought me a number of *gifts*, lessons I might never have received otherwise. They've taken me to dimensions of mental, emotional, social, and spiritual health I've never felt before.

First and foremost I learned to *surrender* and *accept* that as hard as I might try, I am not in control of my life. This is certainly not the first time I've been given this lesson, but it has surely been the most uncomfortable. Bad things do happen to good people, but never accidentally. There's always a reason and something meaningful to learn from them. "OK, I get it now. I truly understand what it means to *let go and let God.* Please God, no more of these lessons. I'm with you. Lead on."

My capacity for *humility*, *compassion*, and *forgiveness* is far greater than it was pre-shingles. I've slowed down, simplified my life, am less angry and fearful (especially of pain), and much to the delight of my wife, a much better listener. Just a few short months ago I found myself fixated on relieving the pain, and now I feel almost overwhelmed with *gratitude*. I'm grateful for simply being alive at this incredibly exciting time and playing a meaningful role in humanity's and the Earth's evolution. I'm eternally grateful for my wife and family, loving friends, and the opportunity to serve others as a healer and teacher.

Perhaps shingles' greatest gift has been the *inspiration* to write this book and help others struggling with chronic pain. Cannabis has been a godsend in both relieving my pain and helping to heal my life. I'm hoping that the following pages will serve you as a guide to your own healing from the plague of chronic pain.

In Part I, I'll provide you with a comprehensive presentation of the most current information on how to use medical marijuana most effectively and safely. Part II will briefly present a state-of-the-art integrative holistic medical treatment for the most common chronic pain conditions (both physical and emotional), using medical marijuana as a complement to the treatment program.

I have treated more than seven thousand chronic pain patients using medical marijuana, and I have reviewed the scientific literature and studies in my quest to develop a standard of care that is both safe and effective. Yet every individual is unique, and reactions can certainly vary to medications, supplements, and medical marijuana. Although there are no known fatalities directly attributable to cannabis, before beginning any new course of treatment, I recommend that you consult with your physician. Keep him or her informed of your progress and report any uncomfortable or adverse side effects that cause you concern.

Remember that the possession and use of cannabis is still illegal under federal law. Neither medical marijuana nor the majority of the supplements recommended in Part II has been evaluated by the Food and Drug Administration. But I can assure you that they are considerably safer than a multitude of pharmaceutical drugs that have been approved by the FDA.

I've changed the names and some identifying details of the patients described in the "Patient Stories" presented in Part II.

In Part III you will learn to integrate cannabis into a holistic approach for self-empowerment, to move beyond temporary pain relief into a life-changing healing process. You'll develop a far greater capacity for practicing exceptional self-care, becoming fully conscious, fully alive, and high on life! Enjoy the journey, dear reader. I'm at your service.

—Dr. Rav

PART I
Cannabis as Medicine

Chapter 1

Marijuana: The Medicine of Empowerment

Through love all pain will turn to medicine.

—Rumi, a thirteenth-century Persian poet, Islamic
scholar, theologian, and Sufi mystic (1207–1273)

What brought you to this book? Maybe you or someone close to you is suffering with the misery—the pure agony—of relentless, severe pain. As you well know, such pain can completely overwhelm your life, to the point where relief from it becomes an all-consuming, single-minded focus. When chronic pain flares and becomes acute, it can immediately extinguish your capacity to enjoy almost anything.

There's no way to soften the blow, rationalize, or negotiate your way around it. Chronic pain is debilitating. When it's severe, it can control our body and mind to the extent that we are totally at its mercy, powerless to stop it.

I know chronic pain. As a physician I have treated chronic pain patients for decades, and as a patient I have been humbled and devastated by the shingles virus.

There is hope, however, for you and others who suffer from chronic pain. With this book, you now have a guide to overcome pain and revitalize your life. There is the very real possibility of feeling better than you ever have. I am offering you the *medicine of empowerment*—the power to regain control and the joy of life that chronic pain has stripped

3

away. And medical marijuana plays a vital role in this self-healing process.

YOU'RE NOT ALONE

Chronic pain affects approximately 100 million people, nearly one-third of our population. More Americans suffer with chronic pain than with diabetes, cardiovascular disease, and cancer *combined*. By necessity (when there is no recognized cure), we are forced to live with painful conditions such as arthritis; low back, knee, neck, or shoulder problems; migraine headaches; irritable bowel syndrome (IBS), acid reflux (GERD), or fibromyalgia; and a host of other uncomfortable problems that never completely resolve. Pain is the number one reason people visit a doctor's office. As a chronic pain sufferer, know that you are not alone.

In addition, it is estimated that nearly 80 percent of our population is plagued with the emotional pain of anxiety and depression, often associated with chronic physical pain.

Whether it is physical or emotional, or it is persistent, recurrent, or incapacitating, chronic pain is humanity's most debilitating disease.

How does today's mainstream medical industry deal with chronic pain? In a word: *opioids*. And with opioids come very real risks, often-times leading to tragedy.

Opioids are narcotic analgesics found in prescription pain relievers such as oxycodone (Oxycontin, Percocet), tramadol, hydrocodone (Vicodin), methadone, fentanyl, meperidine (Demerol), morphine, and codeine. These drugs were developed with the best of intentions, and the vast majority of doctors who prescribe them do so with the best interests of their patients in mind.

But, sadly, the overprescribing, misuse, and abuse of opioids have led to a public health crisis in America. Drug overdose is currently the leading cause of accidental death in the U.S., and opioid addiction is driving this epidemic. In 2014, there were *fifty-two deaths every day from opioid overdose*.

I realize you might be feeling desperate, and opioids may seem like your only option for pain relief. But as many of us know all too well, these drugs can often be minimally effective and highly addictive, and they nearly always cause unpleasant side effects, such as constipation, nausea, drowsiness, and dizziness. And if that's not enough of a deterrent, a study published in June 2016 found that narcotics (specifically morphine) may actually *prolong chronic pain*. There has to be a better way for treating the condition. And this book will provide you with one.

I know exactly what it is like to be in your position. As a patient, when I was suffering from a severe case of shingles, medical marijuana allowed me to gain some control over a seemingly overwhelming situation. While all of my pain did not disappear, marijuana reduced the pain to such an extent that I was not only able to function and work, but could even enjoy my life.

Since 2011, when I opened my current practice, Fully Alive Medicine in Boulder, Colorado, the primary reason patients have come to me is to relieve chronic pain. The vast majority of patients had already been prescribed an opioid, which they were eager to stop taking. After they saw me and began using medical marijuana, I consistently observed a dramatic reduction in their pain, to a point where they were able to either discontinue or, at the very least, substantially reduce their dosage of the prescription narcotics. The same has also been true of the anti-anxiety and antidepressant medications, as well as the sleeping pills often prescribed to chronic pain patients.

Regardless of how long these patients have had their pain, the results of medical marijuana have been remarkable, and in some cases miraculous. When used appropriately it is highly effective, quick, safe, and without any unpleasant side effects.

I promise you, help is on the way. Just as medical marijuana has accompanied me, and thousands of others, on our journey of overcoming chronic pain, and of self-discovery, I now want to share the healing benefits of this wondrous medicinal herb. In the proceeding chapters, I will provide you with all the information you'll need, in addition to serving as your guide for initiating and fully implementing a pain-relieving, transformational, and *re-creational* healing process.

Pain relief is fast and easy, but to heal your life you'll need to address the multiple causes of your ongoing pain—physical, emotional, and spiritual. I'll assist you with this, but it will require your time, persistence, and especially, your commitment. The upside is that you may find it to be the most rewarding work you'll have ever done. I'm here to help you with whatever path you choose for relieving your pain.

EXCEPTIONAL SELF-CARE + CANNABIS = OPTIMAL HEALTH CARE

This book is intended as a guide to using cannabis for:

- Quickly relieving your physical pain
- Creating a treatment program for long-lasting pain relief and for healing your chronic dis-ease (mental, emotional, and spiritual pain)
- Providing a path toward optimal health

You might be thinking, "All I really care about is getting rid of this !*?!* pain!" Or you might ask yourself, "Isn't health the absence of illness? If I'm pain-free, then I'm healthy. Correct?" Not necessarily. The words *health*, *heal*, and *holy*, are all derived from the Anglo-Saxon *haelen*, meaning "to make whole." *Health* is actually a condition of fullness, balance, and wholeness—a sense of being *fully alive!*

The American Board of Integrative Holistic Medicine (ABIHM) defines *holistic* or *optimal health* as the unlimited and unimpeded *free flow of life force energy* through your body, mind, and spirit. It is a state of well-being encompassing physical vitality, mental inspiration, emotional intelligence, an opened heart, and an awakened soul.

The only problem with this definition is that most of us are uncertain about the meaning of the term *life force energy*. "What is it? Have I ever experienced it? How can I consciously create it? What does it feel like?"

The concept of life force energy has been well known for at least five thousand years. It serves as the foundation for traditional Chinese medicine (TCM) and is known as *chi*. In Ayurveda, the traditional medicine of India, it is called *prana*. In Hebrew, life force is *chai*; in Japanese, *ki*; and it is the *tao* in Taoism. The term used by the ABIHM that most closely equates to the feeling generated by this healing energy is *unconditional love*. The primary objective of each of these ancient traditions and disciplines, as well as the practice of holistic medicine, is to strengthen and allow for the free flow of this energy through every aspect of your being. This in turn produces a heightened state of self-awareness and self-love, while greatly enhancing health and a sense of well-being.

I'll be presenting several options for strengthening *chi* and *self-love* throughout the book, especially in Part III. But the primary focus will be on utilizing the one method that has been highly effective throughout recorded history—the holistic medicinal herb *cannabis*.

Our current use of medical marijuana comes with a long legacy of healing. Cannabis has been widely accepted in civilization throughout human history. We find documented use of it in five-thousand-year-old Chinese pharmacology treatises and three-thousand-year-old Ayurveda texts from India, and it is even mentioned in the Bible. In the U.S. it dates back in recorded history to George Washington, who grew hemp at Mount Vernon.

Marijuana, known only as cannabis, was legal for most of American history and was a primary ingredient of the most effective natural remedies for many common ailments, including migraine headache, rheumatism (arthritis), epilepsy, neuralgia (nerve pain), dysmenorrhea (painful menstruation), asthma, depression, insomnia, gastric ulcer, and morphine addiction. Cannabis was introduced into modern medicine in 1839, and shortly thereafter admitted to the *U.S. Pharmacopeia* (USP) in 1851, though for sociopolitical reasons (it had nothing to do with its efficacy or safety), it was de-listed in 1937, *against the advice of the American Medical Association.*

After nearly eighty years of illegality in the U.S., based on specious arguments and inaccurate perceptions, I am pleased to see the progress being made with the re-legalization of cannabis as medicine. It began in 1996 with California, and following the 2016 election, there are now twenty-eight states plus the District of Columbia in which citizens have chosen to legalize medical marijuana. Cannabis is currently ranked fourth among the world's most frequently used substances, behind caffeine, nicotine, and alcohol—all of which are legal, but not one of them has the medicinal properties of cannabis, and except for caffeine, they have significantly greater health risks.

It certainly appears likely that it will not be long before medical marijuana becomes legal in every state. From my perspective as a physician and scientist, there is not and has never been a pharmaceutical drug that possesses its breadth of therapeutic properties.

In those patients choosing to integrate medical marijuana into a holistic medical treatment program, the long-lasting and life-changing results have been extremely impressive. The combination of cannabis and holistic medicine is by far the most consistently successful treatment for a variety of chronic pain conditions I've seen in nearly a half century of practicing the art and science of medicine. I'll present many of these treatment programs in Part II.

MY APPROACH TO HOLISTIC HEALING

I've been a holistic family doctor in Colorado since 1972. My practice grew rapidly during its first decade, but especially after I opened Columbine Medical Center, the first combination family practice/minor emergency center in Colorado (similar to today's urgent care centers). This new model, open thirteen hours a day, seven days a week, quickly became the busiest family practice in the Denver metro area.

This innovative concept was considered a great success. In spite of hiring four other family doctors, I found that the heavy workload took its toll on my health. Seeing a high volume of patients, pressuring myself to stay on time while maintaining quality care and serving as the owner and medical director, literally made me sick. I developed chronic sinusitis.

The word *chronic* is a medical euphemism for *incurable*, but that latter word is rarely used when speaking to a patient. Rather, most patients are given the dismal prognosis, as I was by my ENT (ears, nose, throat) consultant, "You'll have to learn to live with it."

As a patient who'd just been told that I'd have to suffer with the misery of sinus disease for the rest of my life, I instantly felt a combination of hopelessness, grief, fear, and anger. But by the time I got home after leaving my doctor's office, I had transmuted the intense energy of those emotions into a firm commitment to cure the condition: "Whatever is required to do the job of healing my inflamed mucous membrane, I will do it." In spite of not knowing anyone who had been able to do it, I strongly believed I would eventually free myself from the plague of sinus suffering. And eventually, I did!

It took several years and the reclaiming of my holistic medical roots (embedded in osteopathic medicine) before I cured the chronic sinusitis. My holistic treatment program began with dietary changes, and progressed to the daily practice of nasal hygiene and utilizing high-tech indoor-air modification. These changes helped considerably. But it wasn't until I had spent a year working diligently on my mental, emotional, and spiritual health that I achieved my goal. There was no longer any evidence of a sinus problem.

Using marijuana, specifically with the intention of healing my life— i.e., mind (modifying my beliefs and behavior), emotions (identifying, experiencing, and accepting all of my feelings), heart and soul (expanding my capacity to give and receive love and practice forgiveness)—was a key component in this final aspect of my self-healing program.

Having successfully implemented a nonsurgical holistic treatment program to cure the world's most common respiratory condition, I soon realized that a very similar approach (minus the nasal hygiene and air cleaners) could also be applied to any other common chronic condition, from diabetes and heart disease to a wide variety of chronic pain conditions, including arthritis and back pain.

Utilizing all that I had learned during my own healing process, from my holistic colleagues, and from the thousands of patients I had treated as a family doctor, I set out on a new mission—to *transform health care*, while attempting to fulfill my greatest potential as a healer and teacher (*doctor* = Latin for *teacher*). I had regained my passion for medicine and was inspired by the *healing power of love*—the basis of holistic medicine.

In 1987, at the ripe old age of forty, I walked away from conventional medicine and the practice I had birthed and nurtured, leaving what I had once considered the job of my dreams, along with a lifetime of financial security, and started over. My physician father thought I'd lost my mind. With considerable anger, he asked, "You're going to practice what?!"

At the time, I had a strong sense of knowing, a certainty, that the mainstream health care system would inevitably move in this direction, since the holistic approach was far superior to conventional medicine for treating chronic disease. My new job would be training physicians, teaching the public, and helping to establish standards for the art, science, and practice of holistic medicine, based on exceptional self-care and self-love.

Self-love doesn't cost anything. We have access to an infinite supply within each of us (once the mental and emotional obstacles are diminished or removed), and we are the most qualified practitioners to provide this remarkably effective medicine to ourselves. It would have been a no-brainer, but just as with the lack of science regarding the medicinal use of cannabis, the medical community insisted on seeing an abundance of studies that proved the effectiveness of holistic medicine, specifically on the therapeutic benefits of love. Unfortunately there were very few. They needed proof. Fair enough. "In that case," I thought, "heed the advice of Hippocrates: *Physician heal thyself*."

Rather than waiting decades for sufficient convincing documentation of its value, while depriving patients of optimal health care, why not see how a daily megadose of self-nurturing makes you feel and changes your life.

I'm thrilled to be writing this book and sharing with you what I've learned during the past three decades about using cannabis as a holistic medicine for relieving chronic pain and healing your life. The legalization of medical marijuana has helped significantly to facilitate my teaching of holistic medicine. Although it may not be a quick-fix for eliminating all of the causes of your dis-ease, it can certainly help in identifying the multiple factors contributing to your chronic pain. And, most important, it works extremely well for quickly reducing pain, and providing you the space for practicing optimal self-care.

I'm grateful for the opportunity to present what I've found to be the most effective self-healing practices, while imparting the wisdom of Hippocrates. As I continue my thirty-year journey from family doctor to holistic healer, it feels as if I've found the job I've been training for my entire life.

As many of you will find as you read this book, you don't have to be a physician to heal yourself. With good instruction, the implementation of a self-care program along with medical marijuana can be a highly successful strategy for healing, and potentially curing, many common chronic pain conditions. With *Cannabis for Chronic Pain*, you'll learn that *you do not have to live with this misery*. Hopefully you'll also discover a new you in the following pages.

Chapter 2

Getting Started

In August 2016, the Senate passed a bill allowing veterans access to medical marijuana. That same month, the Drug Enforcement Administration (DEA) ruled that marijuana would remain a Schedule 1 controlled substance, which declares that it has "no currently accepted medical use and a high potential for abuse." This keeps the drug in the same category as heroin. Although progress is gradual, we continue to take two steps forward and one step backward in the process of legalizing medical marijuana.

Due to confusion, personal bias, and hidden agendas among politicians and regulatory agencies on the federal and state levels, mixed messages regarding medical marijuana are continuing. This ambiguity creates an atmosphere of insecurity among the public and the medical community that seeks to relieve their pain and suffering. The lack of accurate information regarding the appropriate use of this medicinal herb is significantly impeding progress in greater accessibility for those who can benefit most from it—chronic pain sufferers.

Rather than risk overwhelming you with too much information, I've structured this and the following two chapters in a format of *frequently asked questions*. By providing you with the most basic and necessary information for the safe and effective use of medical marijuana in this way, my intention is to instill a feeling of security and confidence in your capacity to *care for yourself with MMJ* (an often used acronym for medical marijuana). The truth is there are very few other options.

1. What is the difference between hemp and marijuana?

The shift from legal to illegal in 1937 illustrates the degree of confusion that existed, and still exists, between *hemp* and *marijuana*. They're distinguished from each other based on their use. Both come from the same plant—*Cannabis sativa*. The term *hemp* commonly refers to the cannabis *stalk* and *seed* used in industry and commerce for textiles, foods, paper, body-care products, detergents, plastics, and building materials. The term *marijuana* refers to the cannabis flowers smoked or ingested for medicinal, recreational, or spiritual purposes.

2. Is medical marijuana legal in my state, and what are the restrictions?

The following information on the twenty-eight states as well as Washington, DC, that have some form of medical marijuana legalization was last updated in December 2016 by ProCon.org.

States with Medical Marijuana + Possession Limit	
Alaska	1 oz. usable; 6 plants (3 mature, 3 immature)
Arizona	2.5 oz. usable; 12 plants
Arkansas	3 oz. usable per 14-day period
California	8 oz. usable; 6 mature or 12 immature plants
Colorado	2 oz. usable; 6 plants (3 mature, 3 immature)
Connecticut	2.5 oz. usable
Delaware	6 oz. usable
Florida	Amount to be determined
Hawaii	4 oz. usable; 7 plants
Illinois	2.5 oz. of usable cannabis per 14-day period
Maine	2.5 oz. usable; 6 plants
Maryland	30-day supply, amount to be determined
Massachusetts	60-day supply for personal medical use (10 oz.)
Michigan	2.5 oz. usable; 12 plants

Minnesota	30-day supply of non-smokable marijuana
Montana	1 oz. usable; 4 plants (mature); 12 seedlings
Nevada	2.5 oz. usable; 12 plants
New Hampshire	2 oz. usable cannabis during a 10-day period
New Jersey	2 oz. usable
New Mexico	6 oz. usable; 16 plants (4 mature, 12 immature)
New York	30-day supply non-smokable marijuana
North Dakota	23 oz. per 14-day period
Ohio	Maximum of a 90-day supply, amount to be determined
Oregon	24 oz. usable; 24 plants (6 mature, 18 immature)
Pennsylvania	30-day supply
Rhode Island	2.5 oz. usable; 12 plants
Vermont	2 oz. usable; 9 plants (2 mature, 7 immature)
Washington	8 oz. usable; 6 plants
Washington, DC	2 oz. dried; limits on other forms to be determined

As you can see, each state in which medical marijuana is legal has enacted its own set of laws to regulate this industry. The result has been a wide disparity between states that is both disturbing and, in some cases, astounding. For instance, the state of New Jersey, with a population of approximately 9 million, has 5 operating medical marijuana dispensaries in the entire state, while Colorado, with just over 5.5 million people, has 531 medical dispensaries. In the case of New Jersey, the will of the people has apparently been overruled by the politicians, whose primary allegiance appears to be to their benefactors. Not coincidentally, New Jersey is home to several of the world's largest pharmaceutical companies.

Fortunately the Obama administration de-prioritized marijuana prosecutions at the federal level. Since then hundreds of businesses have opened throughout the country to cultivate, distribute, and sell medical cannabis. To learn more about the specific regulations in your state, google "*medical marijuana laws and regulations [your state]*."

3. What are the basic requirements common to all states?

A physician evaluation in order to obtain a medical marijuana license; a qualifying diagnosis (chronic pain is approved in almost all states); and the subsequent purchase of medical marijuana at a licensed medical dispensary or from a licensed caregiver.

4. What are the qualifying diagnoses for an MMJ license?

Other states differ slightly, but in Colorado, medical marijuana may be recommended for the following qualifying medical conditions or for a debilitating medical condition that produces one of the following:

- Severe pain
- Cachexia
- Cancer
- Glaucoma
- HIV or AIDS
- Persistent muscle spasms
- Seizures
- Severe nausea

Before you see a physician to obtain a recommendation for medical marijuana, it is important to know what the qualifying conditions are in your state. Fortunately for most of you, chronic pain qualifies in nearly every state. It is also helpful (and may be required in your state) to bring your medical records supporting the qualifying diagnosis to your initial appointment for the medical marijuana evaluation.

5. If marijuana is now completely legal in my state (i.e., "recreational marijuana"), why should I go to a medical marijuana dispensary instead of a recreational marijuana shop?

Medical marijuana dispensaries are far more likely to have stronger medicinal marijuana products than the recreational shops. This includes strains with a high content of CBD (cannabidiol), which is the strongest pain-relieving cannabinoid. The budtenders—i.e., the employees who assist you in choosing the appropriate marijuana product for your specific chronic pain condition—should be well informed and better trained than their recreational counterparts. The latter are more knowledgeable about the psychoactive products, since that is the intent of the majority of their customers. Sadly, however, a recent study has shown that many of the MMJ budtenders provide incorrect information to their customers. Medical marijuana in the dispensaries is also nearly always the less expensive of the two options, due to the high sales tax levied on recreational marijuana.

6. What is the physician's role?

Physicians generally rely on scientific studies and standard-of-care protocols to guide their delivery of patient care. Since there are relatively few medical cannabis studies and most have not been widely disseminated in medical journals, the vast majority of the physicians who are willing to see patients for a medical marijuana evaluation know very little about maximizing the medicinal properties of cannabis. Many have also tended to have a negative view of medical marijuana as simply a legal means for people to get high.

However, in Colorado this is gradually changing. As more patients take the initiative and obtain MMJ without it being recommended by their primary care physician, an increasing number of doctors see patients who have suffered with chronic pain for years and have experienced a dramatic improvement with medical marijuana. At the same time, many of these patients have either reduced or eliminated their use of prescription drugs, especially opioids, benzodiazepines (for anxiety), antidepressants, and sleep aids. Even without the studies, these impressive results are hard to ignore.

In spite of the growing recognition of MMJ's therapeutic benefits within the medical community of Colorado, a state that has created a model medical marijuana system, there is still a dearth of physicians who can knowledgeably advise their patients on how to best use this remarkable medicine. And if that's the case in Colorado, I'm certain it is also true of every other state that has legalized medical marijuana. This book serves as a guide for the benefit of both medical marijuana patients and the doctors who recommend it.

In meeting the state's requirements for medical marijuana *evaluations*, the role of the physician is to *determine if the patient qualifies as a suitable candidate* for using medical marijuana, and if he or she does, as the office visit is completed, the doctor signs a document issued by the Medical Marijuana Registry (or similar state agency) *recommending* this patient be permitted to use MMJ. (In Colorado, beginning in 2017, this process can be completed online and there is no paper document.) This is *not* a prescription for marijuana. Based on this signed document, the state then issues the patient a medical marijuana license. Known in Colorado as the "*red card*," this permits the cardholder to purchase medical marijuana from a licensed medical dispensary.

The physician guidelines in Colorado for the initial evaluation process of a potential MMJ patient are similar to those for the initial office visit of patients in need of medical treatment other than medical marijuana. This includes an appropriate physical examination, an evaluation of medical and mental health history, as well as pertinent imaging and laboratory data. In many states, including Colorado, patients are required to renew their MMJ license annually.

While these guidelines make good sense from a conventional medical perspective, they do not take into account the relative safety of this medicinal herb, the time required to meet these new guidelines, the fact that most new MMJ patients are already under the care of a primary care physician or specialist, and more important, there is no mention of the need to educate medical marijuana patients on the safe and effective use of this new medicine.

As a cannabis clinician, I and hundreds of other physicians have not had the time to wait for the results of a sufficient number of studies that will take several years to scientifically prove marijuana is helpful for treating chronic pain, anxiety, insomnia, and many other medical problems. Our offices are filled with patients suffering a wide variety of debilitating chronic physical and emotional ailments.

Although they are coming to us for the primary purpose of receiving a physician's recommendation for legally obtaining medical marijuana, as health care providers it would be a formidable challenge to merely sign a document and not also instruct our patients on *how to use MMJ* most effectively for treating their specific condition.

As old patients return annually for a renewal of their MMJ license, or new patients return for a follow-up visit four to six weeks after their initial appointment, *they become our teachers*. Cannabis medicine is not taught in medical school, nor is it likely to be part of the standard medical curriculum anytime soon. Excellent training in this new sub-specialty of holistic medicine can only be obtained from our patients' feedback, cannabis clinician colleagues, conscientious dispensary personnel, a modicum of studies, and through our personal experience with marijuana—medical, spiritual, and recreational.

During the thirty-minute consultations with my medical marijuana patients, I spend the bulk of our time together sharing with them all that I've learned from these various sources. In addition, I educate them on the most effective use of cannabis for treating their specific problem, advising renewing patients on improving their marijuana treatment program and, if any patients are interested, offering recommendations for holistically treating the underlying condition for which they're using medical marijuana.

This book is essentially a comprehensive presentation of the information I would like to offer during consultations with my MMJ patients, if time permitted. The book allows you to digest the material in short segments and at a much more comfortable pace than can be provided in a short office visit.

I can fully appreciate the fact that when it comes to treating a serious health problem, most people prefer a one-on-one in-person consultation with their doctor. But if you're unable to find a good physician within reasonable proximity to your home, through this book I can serve as your self-care guide. If you have questions that are not addressed in the book, you can email me at drrav@fullyalivemedicine.com. I may not be able to respond to every question, but responses to frequently asked questions not included in this book will appear on my website, www.fully alivemedicine.com.

7. How can I find a good doctor?

Ideally you will find a doctor to perform your medical marijuana evaluation who also has expertise for advising you on how to best use the medicine. However, if a physician meeting that description does not exist in your area, you always have the option of using this book, while working with (or without) a local physician to complement it. However, you will need a physician at least to fulfill your state's requirements for a medical marijuana license. These are my recommendations for finding a good doctor:

- Use word-of-mouth referral from someone you trust.
- Google "*MMJ doctor [your city]*"—here you will often find reviews and testimonials from patients.
- Go to www.abihm.org and click on Find an ABIHM Certified Physician. Here you will find the names and locations of more than three thousand holistic physicians (MDs and DOs) who have been *certified by* the American Board of Integrative Holistic Medicine (ABIHM). Botanical (herbal) medicine is one of the components of the core curriculum of integrative holistic medicine. ABIHM-certified doctors practicing in states with legalized medical marijuana would likely be a good choice for an MMJ evaluation as well as for treating your chronic pain condition holistically.

8. How long does it take to receive the MMJ license?

Once you have completed your visit to a physician and have mailed the signed (by the physician) document to the appropriate state agency, your next step is to obtain the medicine. In some states, including Colorado, if you are a *new* MMJ patient, you can take a copy of the signed physician document and a receipt from the post office verifying that it has been mailed (in lieu of the card) and visit a medical dispensary on the same day that you receive your physician evaluation.

If you are renewing your license, it can take from three to six weeks to receive your new card. I'd suggest you see a physician for the renewal evaluation at least a month prior to the expiration date. If you have not yet received your new card within a few days of that date, be sure you have a sufficient supply of medicine to meet your needs for the next three to four weeks.

Beginning in 2017 in Colorado, patients have had the option of having their physician certification completed online. They are still required to have an in-person appointment. But if they choose to (and most patients do), they can ask the physician to complete the certification online at the conclusion of their visit. Patients then fill out their information online, and can expect to receive their license within twenty-four to forty-eight hours.

9. After receiving my MMJ license, how do I obtain the medicine?

There are three ways in which medical marijuana patients can obtain their medicine, depending on the state in which they live—dispensaries, caregivers, and growing their own plants. Visiting a dispensary in close proximity to your home is the most convenient method (similar to visiting your local pharmacy), but there are some states in which this option is not available. You can easily find this information online by googling "*medical marijuana laws [your state]*."

10. What are the criteria for evaluating a dispensary?

To help determine the quality of the dispensary, I ask the following questions:

• Are their plants grown organically and free of pesticides? (Inhaling toxic pesticides can contribute to increased inflammation, thus causing more pain.)

- Have their plants and other products undergone microbiology testing (for bacteria and fungi) as well as analytical chemistry testing to accurately determine cannabinoid content (measured in milligrams—mg), as well as the percentage content of the cannabinoids? (This term will be explained in Chapter 3.)
- Do they have a broad selection of flower, with a variety of indica, sativa, and hybrid strains? How often, if at all, do they have high-CBD strains available for sale?
- How many of the nine different categories of delivery methods described in Chapter 4 do they have available? Most valuable to the chronic pain patient are: *vaporizing* high-CBD hybrids (e.g., Harlequin) and indicas; high-CBD, THCa, and THC-CBD-CBN *tinctures*; hybrid, indica, and high-CBD sublingual and swallowed *tablets*; high-CBD *hash oils* (CO_2-extracted and dispensed in a syringe); hybrid and indica *edibles*; localized (Apothecanna Extra Strength Pain Creme, Mary's Medicinals CBC) and generalized (CBD:THC/1:1 transdermal patch) *topicals*; fresh leaves for *juicing* (these are rarely available) or as an alternative, CBDa and THCa capsules or tinctures.
- If their selection of products is limited, will they accommodate your requests and order the specific products you're looking for?
- How helpful and knowledgeable are the budtenders—i.e., dispensary employees—who interact with and advise their MMJ patient customers?
- How reasonable are their prices? Medical marijuana, with every type of delivery method, tends to be expensive. Prices can vary widely, but as with most other retail items, there are sales and other benefits offered to customers by individual outlets. Most dispensaries in Colorado, for example, offer lower prices to patients who register as a *member* of their dispensary.

By registering as a member, the patient allows the dispensary to grow the six plants that each MMJ patient is permitted by law in Colorado, thus creating a win-win situation. The higher the quality of the dispensary, the more patients will choose to become members. With additional members, the number of plants the dispensary can legally grow is increased, and it is able to provide a broader selection of products to its patients, hire better budtenders, and improve every aspect of its business. The selection of a specific dispensary does not preclude patients shopping elsewhere, but they will not be eligible for member prices there.

11. Who are caregivers?

Most of the states that have legalized medical marijuana have established a system that allows for people who qualify to use marijuana to choose another person to help them grow or acquire it, to sell it directly to the patient, or to advise them how to use it most effectively. These people are referred to as *caregivers*, which is defined as "someone who has agreed to assist with a patient's medical use of marijuana."

Caregivers are not required to have medical or health care qualifications, nor are they necessarily knowledgeable about the therapeutic use of marijuana. But they are generally less expensive than dispensaries. Typically the states with a dispensary system limit the number of patients an individual caregiver may have, so, depending on the state, he or she can help from one person to unlimited numbers of people.

12. What are the caregiver's rights and protections?

After approval by the state Health Department, caregivers are entitled to manufacture or possess medical marijuana in order to provide that medicine to their patients. From then on both the patient and the caregiver are protected from state or local prosecution for possession or cultivation of marijuana, provided it is used for medical purposes and subject to the state's guidelines for allowable quantities (in Colorado the law specifies *no more than two ounces of a usable form of marijuana, and no more than six marijuana plants, with three or fewer being mature, flowering plants that are producing a usable form of marijuana*).

Locating a competent medical marijuana caregiver can be a difficult task. In some states there are organizations associated with the regulatory agency overseeing medical marijuana that can assist you in finding a qualified caregiver.

13. Can I grow my own plants?

If you are unable to find a caregiver and there are no convenient dispensaries (or none at all), you are left with the option of growing your own plants. Some MMJ patients prefer this option in spite of the availability of dispensaries and caregivers.

Medical marijuana patients listed on the Colorado state registry have the right to grow up to six plants themselves. But as you can see from the "Possession Limit" in Table 2.1 above, this can vary widely depending on the state.*

14. How difficult is it to grow marijuana?

I have no expertise on this subject, nor have I ever grown marijuana, but I have heard repeatedly from multiple sources that it is a relatively easy plant to grow. If this is the option you've chosen, then your first step is to identify the specific strains that would be most helpful for treating your condition (you can identify some of these in Chapter 3 and in Part II). For steps two, three, and four—i.e., obtaining the seeds for those strains, the required equipment (for growing indoors), and instructions for growing and harvesting marijuana plants, you will need to search the Internet. There are a multitude of sources for this information.

---

* Those patients who do not inhale and use only edibles, tinctures, cannabis oil, and topicals are able to obtain an extended plant count, since these methods of administration require more plants to produce.

Chapter 3

Understanding the Medicine of Marijuana

Cannabis is a medicinal treasure trove waiting to be discovered.

> —Dr. Raphael Mechoulam, an Israeli organic
> chemist, professor of medicinal chemistry at the
> Hebrew University of Jerusalem, considered the
> "father of cannabis science" (b. 1930)

More than one in three American adults, 35 percent, were given pain-killer prescriptions by physicians in 2015, according to a 2016 report from the Substance Abuse and Mental Health Services Administration. Many of you reading this book were among them. The report also indicates that during 2015 more adults used painkilling prescription drugs than used cigarettes, smokeless tobacco, or cigars combined!

Although these drugs are highly effective for relieving severe acute pain, such as that from serious injuries or postoperative pain, when used for longer than three months to treat *chronic pain*, they are often addictive, cause a multitude of unpleasant side effects, and are sometimes deadly. In 2014, opioids killed nearly 19,000 Americans. That's greater than the total number of Americans murdered that year (15,809). Since 2000 more than 165,000 people have died from prescription pain relievers. These grim statistics indicate the lethal risk and stunning ubiquity of opioids in modern American life, as well as the dramatic increase in the prevalence of chronic pain.

It is extremely frustrating that despite a few good studies demonstrating the effectiveness of cannabis for relieving pain, the Drug Enforcement Administration (DEA) refused to reduce restrictions on marijuana use, maintaining its status as a Schedule 1 controlled substance.

This decision seems to many of us in the medical community to indicate that the DEA is strongly aligned with and protective of the pharmaceutical industry, whose profits are in the billions from opioids alone. When combined with sales of anti-anxiety drugs, sleep medications, and antidepressants, all of which are frequently prescribed to chronic pain patients (most of whom are able to reduce or eliminate pain with medical marijuana), these statistics make it understandable why the drug companies feel so threatened by this remarkable medicinal herb.

In twin studies published in 2016 and April 2017, researchers found that Medicare and Medicaid prescriptions for painkillers, antidepressants, and anti-anxiety medications dropped sharply in states that legalized medical marijuana. The study's authors estimate that because of the reduction in prescribing rates, a nationwide medical marijuana program would save taxpayers about $1.6 billion on Medicare and Medicaid prescriptions annually. Although data include only prescriptions under Medicare and Medicaid, given the totality of the evidence, it seems reasonable to assume that similar patterns hold true for patients on private insurance plans.

Doctors in the Society of Cannabis Clinicians have been reporting for many years that chronic pain patients with access to cannabis reduce their use of opioids by 50 percent on average, and many quit opioids altogether. In my practice, although I don't have an exact figure, I would estimate that the majority are able to stop opioids completely.

By responding to frequently asked questions posed by my patients, I will serve as your guide to the safest and most effective ways to use medical marijuana to relieve your pain and enhance your quality of life.

1. Is marijuana safe?

Yes, it is extremely safe when used appropriately. The greatest health risks of marijuana can be prevented by the following:

a. Avoid smoking any strain of flower or concentrate.

Irritation and chronic *inflammation of the mucous membrane lining the respiratory tract* (nose, sinuses, and lungs) are side effects of smoking. These effects are not specific to high THC content but are true for any strain of cannabis that is *smoked*, and is similar to the effect of smoking cigarettes. This health risk, resulting from direct contact with the smoke, also occurs, but is not as severe, with vaporizing concentrates—e.g., hash oil, wax, and shatter (See Chapter 4). The smoke is generally more harsh (i.e., it produces more "smoke" or visible vapor) than vaporizing the marijuana flower. Although still present to a minimal extent (resulting from dryness and increased urination), the risk of irritation and inflammation to the mucous membrane is even less significant if you *ingest* a high-THC product such as an edible, a tincture, or hash oil. The increased inflammation from smoking can become a contributing factor in chronic sinusitis, nasal allergies, a chronic cough, chronic bronchitis, and lung cancer. These risks appear to be proportional to the amount of cannabis use and the user's predisposition to developing these problems. *Smoking poses the most significant physical risk of cannabis.* This is a chronic adverse physical effect I've observed from nearly four decades of focusing on the treatment of respiratory conditions.

b. Avoid using any high-THC marijuana product on a daily basis.

The following documented *adverse effects* are *chronic* and result from marijuana with relatively *high THC content* that has been *smoked daily*, unless otherwise stated.

- Several studies indicate a link between cannabis use and *psychosis* or *schizophrenia*. (*Psychosis* is defined as a severe mental disorder in which thought and emotions are so impaired that contact is lost with external reality.) This probably represents a *causal* role of cannabis in precipitating the onset of schizophrenia and psychotic episodes. The risk is significant and was most prevalent in adolescents who began smoking in their early teens and continued into early adulthood. The studies also demonstrated that those who persisted in using cannabis reported more persistent psychotic symptoms than those who stopped using cannabis. Psychosis is a major problem, and is by far the *most serious (mental) health risk of chronic marijuana use* (specifically, high-THC strains).

- A large body of evidence demonstrates that cannabis *dependence*, both behavioral and physical, does occur in 7 to 10 percent of regular users, and that early onset of use (adolescence) and especially daily use (of high-THC strains) are strong predictors of future dependence.

- A small but growing body of evidence indicates a significant link between daily use of cannabis and *depression, memory loss, cognitive impairment* (including the inability to discriminate time intervals and space distances), and *information processing*. Depression is associated with low dopamine (a chemical in the body responsible for feelings of pleasure) levels, and *chronic use of marijuana causes the brain to reduce dopamine production.*

- One study showed a connection between cannabis and impaired performance (decreased accuracy and increased response time) on serial addition/subtraction and digit recall tasks. The results of this study suggest that marijuana can adversely affect complex human performance up to twenty-four hours after smoking. If you are smoking on a daily basis, then, performance remains impaired.

c. Adolescents and young adults should avoid using any high-THC marijuana products on a daily basis. The brain is still developing into the mid- to late twenties.

This is by far the *highest risk group for significant adverse mental health effects*, including schizophrenia, abnormal psychosocial development, poor educational outcomes, dependence, and an increased risk of using more harmful and addictive drugs. Education regarding these risks is essentially the only effective preventive measure.

d. Avoid high-THC marijuana products if you have a heart condition.

THC *increases heart rate*, and can also cause postural hypotension (a significant drop in blood pressure when changing positions, e.g., from sitting to standing). But marijuana's cardiovascular effects are not associated with serious health problems for most healthy users.

Cannabis has occasionally caused heart attacks and strokes, but only in people with preexisting cardiovascular disease.

e. Avoid high-THC marijuana products if you are prone to higher levels of anxiety.

   Psychologically and emotionally, THC may induce unpleasant reactions such as *anxiety*, disconnected thoughts, panic reactions, disturbing changes in perception, paranoia, delusions, and hallucinatory experiences. This is especially true in people who already have a predisposition toward higher levels of anxiety.

f. Other health effects include:

   - Within twenty-four hours of using a high-THC product (after the psychoactive effect has dissipated), most people will experience some degree of *irritability*, *fatigue*, and possibly mild *depression*. This is to some extent a "rebound" from the euphoria and energizing effect of THC, along with a compensatory reaction of the brain to reduce dopamine release.
   - Marijuana causes dry mouth, nose, and eyes, due to decreased blood flow to the periphery of the body and increased blood flow through the kidneys, resulting in increased urination. *Drink* lots of water to counter this drying effect.
   - Marijuana can also increase urinary obstruction in men over fifty with preexisting BPH (benign prostatic hyperplasia). This results in increased urinary frequency and urgency.

   There have been rare cases of someone committing suicide after eating far too much of an edible, however researchers have not found even one death directly attributable to marijuana.

   Although the risk of schizophrenia is not great, I've seen how devastating it can be to both the afflicted person as well as his or her family. One of my patients described in detail the story of her twenty-two-year-old daughter who had been a perfectly healthy, bright, and highly functioning adolescent and young woman until shortly after graduating from college. Within the space of three to four weeks her mental health rapidly deteriorated to the point where she lost touch with reality, suffered a severe psychotic episode, and was admitted to a psychiatric hospital.

There was no family history of schizophrenia, but after hearing more of her history, I was able to speculate on the multiple factors contributing to her illness. It cannot be proven, but I strongly suspect that this was a case of cannabis-induced schizophrenia, triggered by a series of traumas throughout her life.

Although in this case there were other notable factors in addition to the daily use of sativa (high-THC) strains, who among us did not experience major emotional stress at some point during late adolescence and early adulthood? It's easy and quite tempting for a young person to avoid confronting these issues and doing the difficult emotional work, while making problems "disappear" by smoking marijuana. But after this temporary euphoria dissipates, adolescents are right back where they started, with possibly even worse anxiety and depression.

Even though this same reaction can also occur in older adults using high-THC products as an escape from feeling painful emotions, the fragility of the developing adolescent brain makes psychosis from cannabis a far greater concern. In this younger age group, if a high-THC strain is smoked daily with the *intention* of quickly relieving emotional pain, it can potentially become a serious problem. *Schizophrenia*, a form of psychosis, is undoubtedly the *greatest mental health risk of THC*.

2. Is marijuana addictive?

Any substance or behavior that affects the "reward system" of the brain, including food, sex, and even television, and directly or indirectly affects dopamine metabolism, has the potential for dependence and possible addiction.

Although popular belief implies otherwise, *marijuana can be addictive*. Marijuana use can lead to the development of problem use, known as a *marijuana use disorder*, which in severe cases takes the form of addiction. To avoid misunderstanding, it is important to distinguish *addiction* from chronic use, problem use, recreational use, and medicinal use.

According to the American Society of Addiction Medicine, *addiction* is defined as "a primary, chronic disease of brain reward, motivation, memory, and related circuitry. Dysfunction in these circuits leads to characteristic biological, psychological, social, and spiritual manifestations. This is reflected in an individual pathologically pursuing reward and/or relief by substance use and other behaviors.

"Addiction is characterized by inability to consistently abstain, impairment in behavioral control, craving, diminished recognition of significant problems with one's behaviors and interpersonal relationships, and a dysfunctional emotional response."

Marijuana differs from far more addictive drugs, such as cocaine and heroin, because these have a more pronounced ability to affect this reward system more quickly, and there are increased potency and lethality associated with the side effects of cocaine and heroin, including respiratory depression, hypoxia, cardiac arrest, overdose, and death.

In 2014, 4.176 million people in the U.S. abused or were dependent on marijuana, and 138,000 voluntarily sought treatment for their marijuana use. Research has clearly demonstrated that people who begin using marijuana before the age of eighteen are four to seven times more likely than those who start as adults to develop problem use. Dependence becomes addiction when the person can't stop using marijuana even though it interferes with his or her daily life. Studies suggest that 9 percent of people who use marijuana will become dependent on it, and this rises to about 17 percent in those who start using in their teenage years. These are similar to the number of people that can become addicted to other drugs such as alcohol, cocaine, or opiates. Addiction can cause a host of problems in daily life, especially maintaining a job or relationships.

Although marijuana is less harmful than alcohol, cocaine, and opiates, any drug that affects the brain reward system in the *vulnerable individual* can lead to problem use, dependence, and in severe cases, addiction. In most *cases* of addiction, *it is not the drug, but the user of the drug that is the major contributor to causing addiction.* Careful attention to an individual's mental health history, such as a diagnosis of addiction, depression, anxiety, or a mood disorder, or a family history of addiction, should serve as a warning to the possibility of marijuana being a potential problem. Does the benefit outweigh the risk? These factors need to be taken into account before beginning daily cannabis use for chronic pain, and should be discussed with your physician.

Behavioral support has been effective in treating marijuana addiction. No medications are currently available to treat it.

Marijuana potency has steadily increased over the past two decades. THC content increased from 3.7 to 7.5 percent in the early 1990s to 9.6 to 16 percent in 2013. With the advent of THC concentrates, such as *shatter* and *wax* (see Chapter 4), the addiction potential of marijuana has increased considerably. The highest-potency marijuana *flower* available today contains at most 25 to 30 percent THC. But the concentrates can contain up to *95 percent or more THC.* The effect is so intense and the addiction potential so much greater that they have been described as the "crack cocaine of marijuana."

Researchers do not yet know the full extent of the consequences when the body and brain (especially the developing brain) are exposed to extremely high concentrations of THC or whether the recent increases in emergency department visits by people testing positive for marijuana are related to rising potency. I believe the risk of dabbing and the use of strong concentrates, e.g., shatter and wax, far outweighs their benefit, especially in late adolescence and early adulthood. *I strongly advise my patients to avoid them.*

3. Can I use marijuana and go to work?

There are many variables to consider in responding to this question. Your degree of pain, your level of functionality with the specific marijuana product you're planning to use, the nature of your work, and your employer's rules and regulations are some of the primary considerations.

Each of us is unique and will respond a bit differently to marijuana. As you'll learn in question 5, the marijuana products most effective for relieving pain are not strongly psychoactive, and the effect of the THC in them is mitigated by both CBD and the pain itself. Many of my chronic pain patients, especially those who are self-employed or who work from home, are able to function and perform their jobs well while medicating with marijuana. The majority of those employed outside the home, however, refrain from inhaling or ingesting medical marijuana during work hours, and wait until they leave their workplace.

Those who do use MMJ while at work will often use either a topical cream (see "Topicals" in Chapter 4) without any THC (and no psychoactive effect), or a high-CBD tincture or hash oil with minimal amounts of THC. A transdermal patch is another possibility (see Chapter 4). It's discreet, and if you find it's adversely affecting your job performance, you can peel it off and the effect will dissipate within a half hour.

I suggest you test yourself on the weekend or a non-working day by taking the product you're considering using during work and seeing how it affects you. If it's too strong—i.e., too psychoactive— then try a smaller dose. Tinctures provide an excellent method for determining your ideal dose.

4. Can I drive a car while under the influence of marijuana?

There is an increased risk of motor vehicle accidents, although this risk is not nearly as significant as with alcohol. Drivers under the influence of marijuana were found to drive more slowly, while those intoxicated with alcohol drove faster. This risk can be prevented by simply avoiding driving within three to four hours after smoking or vaporizing.

5. Do I have to get high to benefit from medical marijuana?

The short answer is *NO*. But to relieve chronic pain, this medicine is most effective when there is some THC present.

There are a small minority of patients who would prefer not to experience any psychoactive effect, commonly referred to as getting high. I've been told emphatically by a few patients who were applying for a new medical marijuana card and had little or no prior experience, "I don't want to get high." Some of these people had used marijuana recreationally years before and had an unpleasant experience, resulting in high anxiety or paranoia, and never used it again. Others were simply afraid of the unknown or of "being out of control," and were aware that it's because of the psychoactive effect that marijuana had been deemed unsafe and still remains federally illegal. Although these are valid concerns, once patients are better informed about the quality and consistency of medical marijuana products and how to best use them for their specific problem, and have a better understanding of what an altered state of consciousness is and how it can be used beneficially, the majority of them are willing to try the treatment.

The psychoactive effect is generally only a "problem" with high-THC strains of marijuana, which are too strong for many people and *not recommended for treating chronic pain*. I've also noticed that when patients use products containing significant amounts of THC (20 to 25 percent THC) for treating more severe pain—i.e., above a pain level of a 5—the psychoactive effect is somewhat mitigated. You will not feel as high as if you had taken this same product at a time when you were experiencing little or no pain.

Researchers have not yet been able to explain how it occurs, but it's evident that *THC activates and significantly enhances the analgesic effect of CBD (cannabidiol)*, considered the most potent pain reliever of all the cannabinoids. CBD is not psychoactive.

We now have the benefit of more than twenty years of accumulated data from clinical experience and feedback from MMJ patients, along with increasingly more accurate laboratory analysis. What we've found is that *high-CBD products with negligible amounts of THC will relieve pain, but not as dramatically as those with a higher THC content*. However, these same products are more effective for reducing anxiety than those with higher amounts of THC. In those people who are normally more anxious, THC will often *increase their anxiety* and possibly keep them awake at night. And as most of you are aware, *when you are more anxious or sleep deprived, your pain is worse.*

When CBD is combined with THC, which is the case with the most effective medical marijuana products for relieving pain, it will significantly *reduce the psychoactive effect*, but the effect will not be eliminated. If you've been taking prescription opiates for pain, you will most likely be able to reduce your dosage by using high-CBD products. But eliminating these drugs entirely, as most of my chronic pain patients have been able to do, will usually require a medical marijuana product with significantly higher amounts of THC—e.g., those with a CBD:THC ratio of 1:1, 2:1, or 3:1. And, as a side effect, you will to some extent get high.

The psychoactive effect can also be reduced by taking citicoline, a popular brain supplement, *before* using an MMJ product with a significant amount of THC. One of the main benefits of citicoline is that it increases the level of acetylcholine within the brain. This is a neurotransmitter that plays a vital role in the development and formation of memory and a number of other cognitive processes. Citicoline can be found in most health food stores.

For those patients with chronic pain who remain steadfast in their resistance to experiencing even a mild high, the *psychoactive effect can be avoided* by taking CBD-hemp oil containing almost no THC (I'll explain more about this in question 11). But be aware, it is not as effective an analgesic as those products containing THC.

Given all of these variables, determining the right product and dosage for you will entail a brief process of experimentation to see how you respond and how much of a high is acceptable to you.

6. What is THC?

THC (delta-9-tetrahydrocannabinol) is the first-discovered, most psychoactive, and best known of the more than eighty cannabinoids found in cannabis. Since it binds to the CB1 receptors found predominantly in the brain, THC produces what patients refer to as a "head high"—i.e., it primarily affects your mind, rather than your body. Recognized and appreciated most for its pleasurable psychoactive effect, THC also contains a great number of holistic (whole-person) medicinal benefits. These include:

- Happiness
- Increased energy
- Sensory enhancement
- Pain relief
- Anti-emetic effects (reduces nausea and vomiting)
- Anti-cancer effects
- Anti-inflammatory effects
- Appetite stimulation
- Relief for glaucoma and autoimmune disorders, especially multiple sclerosis

THC when isolated and used *alone* is mildly effective for relieving pain. A good example is the prescription drug Marinol, which consists only of synthetic THC. But when inhaled or ingested in its natural state in combination with other cannabinoids and terpenes (organic compounds found in cannabis, many with medicinal properties—see question 10 below), THC can become a far more powerful analgesic. This is referred to as the *entourage effect*.

Prior to the legalization of medical marijuana in California in 1996, marijuana was used almost exclusively for getting high, and nearly all of the available illegal marijuana had a high THC content, although not as much as we find today. These plants contained very little CBD, and were therefore lacking in many of the therapeutic benefits found in our currently far more sophisticated cannabis medicine chest.

7. How do you know if you're high, and how can it help you if you are?

The THC in marijuana blocks inhibitory neurotransmitters (brain chemicals) whose purpose is to block the release of dopamine, a neurotransmitter responsible for producing feelings of pleasure. This allows an unmitigated flow of dopamine and subsequent feelings of intense pleasure, a major component of the psychoactive effect.

Many of my chronic pain patients have reported to me, "I'm not really sure if the THC is doing anything directly to relieve the pain, but it sure takes my mind off of it." And therein lays the essence of the psychoactive effect of THC. Getting high simply means a *higher level of consciousness*, frequently accompanied by higher levels of *happiness* and *energy* (patients often report, "I can get a lot done while I'm high"). With intention, it can shift you into an experience of the spiritual properties of cannabis. This translates into a *deeper awareness* of: your body (*Where does it feel restricted, uncomfortable, or painful?*); your thoughts and beliefs (*What critical, limiting, or negative messages do I repeatedly give myself that often precipitate higher levels of anxiety, which then increase the pain? What creative ideas come to mind that excite and inspire me?*); your emotions (*What am I feeling? What thoughts, situations, or images trigger fear, anger, sadness, joy, or pain?*); your surroundings (*What inherent beauty in my environment have I been overlooking?*); the people with whom you share your life (*Who consistently causes me pain and depletes my energy, and from whom do I feel support and acceptance and feel energized?*); and your soul (*What warms my heart, feels nurturing and compassionate, elicits joy, or feels like fun?*).

For at least a couple of hours of *expanded awareness*, if it is your intention to do so, it is possible to step back from your pain, to see yourself and your life while experiencing your present reality from *your soul's perspective*. This is called *witness consciousness*.

Many spiritual teachers define *soul* as your *true* or *higher self*, or your connection to God. However you describe it, under the influence of cannabis in a somewhat altered state, and if it is your desire to do so, you can gain a greater measure of *soul awareness*. You experience soul as separate from, yet interwoven with, your body and mind, and it serves you as a *nurturing guide in the practice of self-compassion*. This realization alone can be profoundly healing.

The experience of being high can also be quite pleasurable. If you allow the space for this life energy to flow (some *alone time* is recommended for this), it can be a sensory delight, encompassing a heightened sense of vision, hearing, smell, taste, touch, and intuition. Enhanced creativity, playfulness, and laughter are often part of a psychoactive experience. If shared with a spouse, partner, or lover, it will often deepen your heart connection. It is not frightening. You are simply expanding the breadth and depth of your awareness. Instead of your usual state of *doing* and *thinking*, this is a state of relaxed vitality that shifts you into more of a *being* and *feeling* mode. Don't worry, you won't turn into a vegetable and stop doing and thinking. But at least for two to three hours you will have a better understanding of the term "human *being*," and what is needed for you to lead a more balanced life.

This is a very brief explanation of why THC can potentially be such a powerful and pleasurable holistic medicine as well as a sacred herb, one that has been used for thousands of years as a catalyst for *spiritual awakening*. I'll present this subject in more depth in Chapter 16, "Cannabis as a Sacred Herb."

These therapeutic and pleasurable effects I've described for THC are not experienced by everyone who uses it. I have spoken with several patients, probably less than 5 percent, who *do not find THC and the psychoactive effect to be pleasurable or energizing*. Some have mentioned fatigue as a side effect, and others feel anxious or even a bit depressed.

Remember that each of us is unique and will therefore react somewhat differently. There are also the variables of strain specificity and dosage. What are you using and how much did you take? I recommend at least a two- to three-week trial period to accurately determine whether MMJ is beneficial for you.

8. What are the side effects from THC?

The *physical* effects (other than psychoactive) of THC result in part from its properties as a central vasodilator—i.e., it dilates or opens the arteries flowing through the brain, heart, and kidneys—and a peripheral vasoconstrictor—i.e., it constricts or narrows blood flow to the periphery of the body, such as the skin, fingers, toes, and even your nose and eyes.

What you'll notice if you pay attention to what's happening to your body and mind shortly after using an MMJ product with a high

THC content—e.g., a sativa strain of flower or a high-THC tincture, edible, or concentrate—are the following *acute* effects:

- The experience of getting high—from the heightened flow of dopamine and increased arterial blood flow to your brain, which in turn allows for more of the THC to interact with the CB1 receptors in the brain (you will often lose track of time)
- Increased heart rate—from increased blood flow to your heart
- Increased urination—from increased blood flow to your kidneys
- Increased thirst and dry mouth, nose, and eyes—from increased urination together with decreased blood flow to your mouth, the mucous membrane lining your nose, and your conjunctiva (the surface or outermost layer of your eyeball)
- Increased appetite
- Increased tendency to sunburn—because of decreased blood flow to your skin making it more vulnerable to the sun, even if you have a dark complexion

To maintain comfort and to counterbalance these effects, while maximizing the healing benefits of THC, I recommend doing the following:

- Drink lots of water and make sure you have convenient access to a bathroom.
- Avoid strenuous aerobic exercise in order to prevent tachycardia (abnormally rapid heart rate)—mild to moderate exercise is usually fine.
- Use a saline nasal spray and appropriate eyedrops for dry nose and eyes.
- Apply sunscreen and use sunglasses if you're outdoors.
- Give yourself at least two hours of alone time and include journaling as part of the experience, unless you're with others who are using marijuana recreationally.

9. What is the difference between the sativa and the indica strains?

In 2017, the major classifications of *marijuana flower* (also known as *weed* or *bud*) are *sativa*, *indica*, and *hybrid*. (However, I believe this classification system will change in the near future, as we learn more about terpenes and their therapeutic effects.) Sativa strains tend to be more energizing and mind-stimulating, while the indicas are more for relaxing, for a body high. Sativas are tall-growing, gangly plants, with very narrow leaves; and indicas are shorter, bushier, stay lower to the ground, are better able to survive colder weather, and are more productive.

The *sativa* or *indica* designation can also indicate the *dominance of each specific strain with respect to THC*. As a general rule (and there are exceptions to every rule), sativas have higher amounts of THC (from 5 to 30 percent) than are found in indica, while indica strains typically have lower amounts of THC and a higher CBD content than you would usually find in a sativa.

However, every strain of marijuana, regardless of its dominance as either sativa or indica, is to varying degrees, a *hybrid*. This means there is always a combination of several cannabinoids (and terpenes) present. For example, every indica strain has some THC present, and depending on the amount, you may experience some degree of psychoactivity. But when a strain is labeled as "hybrid," it generally means it is relatively close to a 50:50 or 60:40 ratio.

The degree of dominance is typically noted by a ratio of sativa:indica (in S-dominant strains) or indica:sativa (in I-dominant strains), which is often clearly marked on the labels of the jars in which the plant is stored on the counter of medical marijuana dispensaries. A plant with a ratio of 70:30 or higher (S:I or I:S) is considered to be either sativa or indica, whichever is the 70 percent component, and is no longer labeled a hybrid.

However, these ratios can vary for the same strain. For example, a popular sativa strain is Golden Goat, which usually has an S:I ratio of 70:30. But depending on where and how it was grown, and the laboratory in which it was tested, there are also strains of Golden Goat that are 60:40/S:I. Although there are discrepancies, nearly all strains with the same name will remain in their category of dominance (either sativa or indica) and test very close to the same ratio (as this example demonstrates), whether they are grown in Colorado, California, or another state. For this reason, it is very helpful to pay attention to the name of the specific strain you're using and make note of how it affects you. As you will soon learn, given the complexity of the herb, no two sativas or indicas will have exactly the same effect, even if they are the same ratio.

10. What are cannabinoids and terpenes?

Medical and recreational marijuana, as well as hemp, all stem from the same plant—*Cannabis sativa*. A highly complex herb, cannabis is home to at least eighty different *cannabinoids* and more than one hundred *terpenes*. Each strain of marijuana has a unique combination of cannabinoids and terpenes, and will therefore affect each of us a bit differently. As research continues, the number of identified cannabinoids and terpenes is likely to increase. Each of these substances found in marijuana, the flower of the cannabis plant, has multiple properties, the majority of which are still unknown. However, of those cannabinoids that have already been identified and studied, nearly all have been found to be *medicinal*. Even less is known about terpenes, but this is rapidly changing and the study of these aromatic chemicals is the next frontier of cannabis research.

There are approximately twenty thousand terpenes in the plant kingdom, but very little is known about their medicinal effects. However, due to their presence in cannabis, they have been the focus of recent research. In 2016, some researchers concluded that the *terpenes may be the critical ingredient determining whether the strain is indica or sativa, and not the amount of THC.* However, more research is needed before a definitive conclusion is reached. But from the findings that have already been documented, the terpene myrcene seems to have the most powerful impact on the ultimate effect of the different strains of marijuana. In addition to its being described as a *potency multiplier*, myrcene can also help to determine whether the strain is sedating (indica—if it contains more than 0.5 percent myrcene) or energizing (sativa—if the strain contains less than 0.5 percent myrcene). We also have learned that several of the terpenes serve as both a complement to the medicinal cannabinoids and to some extent an enhancement to the psychoactive effect.

The most distinctive quality of terpenes is their odor, which imparts a beneficial aromatherapy effect to the user. For example, the terpene limonene has a citrus odor, which can elevate mood, reduce anxiety and heartburn, and be used as an antifungal, antibacterial, and anticarcinogenic agent.

It will take additional funding and several years of cannabis research before we definitively determine the beneficial qualities of each of these approximately two hundred chemical compounds. Currently, laboratory analysis of the medical marijuana sold in the majority of dispensaries includes neither the terpene content nor many of the cannabinoids that are present in very small amounts. Only those cannabinoids with the highest content and known medicinal effects are measured.

Of all the cannabinoids that have been identified, THC and CBD are the two with which the public, dispensaries, and researchers are most familiar and for which we have the most information regarding benefits and health risks.

11. Is CBD a good choice for me?

CBD (cannabidiol) is not psychoactive but is currently among the most medicinal and safest of all the cannabinoids. Studies, together with clinical experience, have demonstrated the following therapeutic properties:

- Analgesic (pain-relieving)
- Anti-inflammatory
- Anxiolytic (reduces anxiety and helps relieve post-traumatic stress disorder—PTSD)
- Sleep-inducing
- Antiemetic (reduces nausea and vomiting)
- Muscle relaxant (reduces muscle spasms associated with multiple sclerosis, paralysis, and cerebral palsy and the tremors of Parkinson's)
- Anticonvulsant (decreases both frequency and intensity of seizures in both children and adults)
- Antipsychotic

- Anticancer
- Improves blood circulation
- Lowers blood pressure
- Antidiabetic (lowers blood sugar)
- Helps relieve autoimmune disorders
- Stimulates bone production
- Antioxidant (helps relieve the severity of symptoms with neurodegenerative disorders, such as MS and Parkinson's)
- Antibacterial
- Reduces prostate enlargement and frequency of nighttime urination—not scientifically documented but consistently observed by myself and several patients

There is no other medicinal herb, or pharmaceutical drug, that possesses such a wide array of therapeutic applications. Many patients refer to the effects of CBD as conveying a *body high*—i.e., a feeling of deep physical relaxation without an altered mental state. The fact that it is perfectly safe makes it a highly appealing medicine. A 2011 review published in *Current Drug Safety* concludes that CBD "does not interfere with psychomotor and psychological functions" (as does THC). The authors add that several studies suggest that CBD is "well tolerated and safe" even at high doses. Most of this evidence comes from animals, since very few studies on CBD have been carried out in human patients.

Numerous studies suggest that CBD also *mitigates the THC high*, reducing both memory impairment and paranoia. And as with THC, CBD has been found to present no risk of lethal overdose.

Tolerance, which means that higher doses are required to achieve the same benefits over time, often occurs with products containing higher amounts of THC, but *not* with CBD. In fact, there appears to be some *reverse tolerance* in that users can *reduce* the dose of CBD by 50 to 75 percent while maintaining the same benefits. In addition, CBD appears to reduce the tolerance of opioids and other drugs, meaning a decrease in those drug requirements. The mechanism appears to be the modulation of opioid receptors rather than any change in drug levels of those substances. Also observed with CBD are reductions in addictive symptoms from opioids, as well as reductions in withdrawal effects for opioids, nicotine, and benzodiazepines.

A pharmaceutical version of CBD was recently developed by a drug company based in the UK. The company, GW Pharmaceuticals, is now funding clinical trials on CBD as a treatment for schizophrenia and certain types of epilepsy. It would certainly be ironic if it were found to be effective for treating schizophrenia, which, as I've previously mentioned, can potentially be the most harmful side effect of THC.

What I've learned during the past six years, from listening attentively to my patients' stories and obtaining feedback from conscientious dispensary personnel and cannabis clinician colleagues, as well as from treating my own case of shingles, is that *the combination of the cannabinoids CBD and THC is the safest and most potent pain-relieving medicine in existence.*

CBD acts as an ideal complement to THC, creating a synergistic therapeutic effect. *Together they serve as a powerful analgesic* with a reduced psychoactive effect. The THC appears to activate the CBD, enhancing its analgesic effect. This explains why the *products* (e.g., tinctures) *with a CBD:THC ratio of 1:1, 2:1, or 3:1 are most effective for pain.* Though they aren't exactly comparable to 1:1/CBD:THC, *strains of marijuana flower with a ratio of 50:50 or 60:40/indica: sativa or 60:40/sativa:indica have a similar high pain-relieving potency.* The ratios of CBD:THC or indica:sativa are found on the labels of most MMJ products.

Although it is most frequently used for pain relief, reducing anxiety, and relieving insomnia, CBD has received a great deal of publicity in recent years as a result of its anticonvulsant properties, especially in children. In an August 2013 CNN broadcast, Dr. Sanjay Gupta reported being a skeptic about medical marijuana until he saw the evidence regarding the effectiveness of CBD for dramatically reducing seizures in children. This report resulted in numerous families moving to Colorado to gain access to high-quality CBD for their children with severe and disabling seizure disorders (often with more than one hundred seizures per day).

In my practice, by far the most frequent uses of CBD are for treatment of chronic pain, insomnia, and especially anxiety. Since the focus of this book is on chronic pain, both physical and emotional, I will not be discussing CBD's application in treating seizures, other than to report that it appears to be highly effective in reducing the frequency and intensity of seizures for both adults with epilepsy and, especially, children with the most severe and incapacitating seizure disorders.

I have personally seen very few patients who have used CBD *alone* (without any or with less than 1 percent THC), who have found it to be as effective an analgesic for chronic pain as when it is used in conjunction with some THC. Although not as strong, it still relieves pain and has been reported to work well by a growing number of clinicians and patients (including many former and active NFL players).

With the rapidly increasing demand for CBD, growers have been developing a number of new high-CBD strains of both indica and sativa. In addition to Harlequin and Cannatonic, which have been in existence for several years, other examples of high-CBD strains are: Charlotte's Web, Otto, Haley's Hope, Lucy, Cannatsunami, Strawberry Cookie, and Remedy. These strains (and there are many more) are often used to make high-CBD tinctures, oils, edibles, topicals, and transdermal patches; or they can be vaporized or smoked.

12. What specific strains are best for relieving pain?

As the medical marijuana industry has grown, it has rapidly been adjusting to meet the increasing need for more effective pain products (i.e., *higher amounts of CBD combined with THC*). As a result, marijuana growers have developed a multitude of new strains, many of which are approximately 50:50/S:I, but some of which are 60:40/I:S (indica-dominant) and 60:40 or 70:30/S:I (sativa-dominant). I have listed the *most effective strains for relieving pain* below.

Pay close attention to the strains you use and maintain a record of their impact on your pain and anxiety (sativas have a tendency to increase anxiety, and indicas to reduce it). For example, if your pain is reduced from a 7 to a 3, you can very simply make a note such as *Harlequin: Pain* ↓ *7* → *3; Anxiety* ↓ *5* → *2* (you can use the "MMJ Log" in the Introduction to Part II to record your reactions). In doing this you can easily determine which strains work best for you, while also rotating the most effective strains. It is important to rotate three or four different strains (don't use the same one every day) to avoid developing a tolerance to one strain.

I'm not sure where the names of these strains came from, but they are certainly easy to remember. Here are some examples of the most effective, popular, and available *hybrids* (all are close to 50:50/S:I) for pain. The names are universal, and the strains should be similar regardless of the state in which they're grown.

- Agent Orange
- AK-47
- Biodiesel
- Blue Dream
- Don Shula
- Gorilla Glue
- Harlequin (in addition to being 50:50/S:I, it also has a very high CBD content; one of the most effective MMJ products for quickly relieving pain)
- Lemon Kush
- Mango Kush
- Pineapple Express
- Sage
- Skywalker OG
- Trainwreck
- White Widow

Among the indica-dominant 60:40s and 70:30s are:

- Afghan Kush
- Banana Kush
- Blackberry Kush
- Blueberry
- Bubba Kush

- Cotton Candy Kush
- Ghost OG
- Girl Scout Cookie
- Lucy (a 70:30 indica, especially high in CBD)
- Master Kush
- Northern Lights
- OG Kush
- Purple Kush
- Tea Tree

Included in the sativa-dominant 60:40s and 70:30s are:

- Bruce Banner
- Chem-4
- Chemdawg
- Chocolope
- Durban Poison
- Golden Goat
- Headband
- Jack Herer
- Lemon Haze
- Maui Wowie
- NYC Diesel
- Red Dragon
- Sour Diesel
- Super Silver Haze

This is by no means a complete list, and the availability of these hybrids depends on the dispensary. What these strains all have in common is their *effectiveness for quickly relieving pain*. Depending on your sensitivity, some of the sativas might make you too high or too anxious, while some of the indicas may cause you to feel too sleepy during the day. However, if you're keeping a record of what strains you've used and what effect they had on you, you will be able to choose the appropriate strain. It's best to initially test a new strain at a time when you have two to three hours in which you are relatively free from any work-related or personal responsibilities. Remember to rotate several strains (three or four similar potency strains) and not use the same strain for more than three consecutive days, to avoid developing a tolerance. It's also helpful for health reasons (especially if you're smoking), and secondarily to lessen tolerance, to periodically vary the method of administration (see Chapter 4).

The ratio of each of these strains may vary to a minimal extent depending on where and how it was grown. For instance, one of the most popular strains of marijuana in Colorado is Blue Dream. Generally considered a 50:50 hybrid, on occasion it will test as a 60:40 sativa-dominant strain.

All strains of indica flower are to some extent hybrids—i.e., they always contain both CBD and THC, but usually with higher amounts of CBD and lower amounts of THC than are typically found in sativa strains. This is the reason most indica strains are more effective for relieving pain than the stronger sativas—i.e., those above an S:I ratio of 60:40. CBD reduces both pain and anxiety, and as most of you are aware, *the greater your anxiety the higher your pain level*. The higher THC strains tend to increase anxiety.

Those patients suffering with chronic pain who can tolerate only a mild psychoactive effect should use only indica strains of 70:30/I:S or higher. In most instances, this will provide them with higher CBD content along with enough THC to activate the CBD and produce only a mild high. Although these strains will reduce the pain, they are not quite as effective as those with a higher percentage of THC.

I also recommend these stronger indica strains for treating *anxiety* and *insomnia*, since THC can potentially increase anxiety and keep patients awake. With higher CBD accompanied by *minimal amounts of THC*—i.e., the stronger indica strains—anxiety is diminished and sleep enhanced. Those strains most effective for anxiety, depending on its severity, have an indica:sativa percentage ratio of 70:30 or 80:20. For sleep and severe anxiety, I recommend the strongest indicas, those with the least amount of THC, 80:20 or higher, and sometimes a 70:30 if it's high in CBD content, e.g., Lucy.

Besides those that involve vaporizing or smoking the flower, there are a number of other high-CBD products, such as tinctures, concentrates, edibles, tablets, and transdermal patches, that are also highly effective for relieving pain. I'll be discussing these in greater depth in the following chapter.

Patients with PTSD and high anxiety levels are able to use the heavy indicas and high-CBD products during the day without getting sleepy. But if you are not someone prone to higher levels of anxiety, the 80:20 and even 70:30 strains might make you feel a bit sedated if used during the day. I've heard many of my patients refer to this feeling as "couch-lock," and they complain "I can't get anything done." This may be the *only significant adverse effect of CBD*. But it is easily avoided by not using a strong indica or high-CBD product during daytime hours.

CBD, when used alone or with minimal THC, is a mild to moderate pain reliever. For those chronic pain patients who *do not want to feel* any *psychoactive effect*, there are currently several options of *CBD oil* with less than 1 percent THC. These might be labeled 20:1 or 25:1/CBD:THC if obtained in an MMJ dispensary, or have no mention of THC if purchased as "CBD hemp oil" in a retail store or online.

13. Is CBD legal?

The answer depends on where it originated. Cannabidiol (CBD) comes in two main forms and is grown for different purposes. CBD can be produced from medical marijuana plants or from industrially grown hemp plants. As I mentioned in Chapter 2, question 1, both are varieties of cannabis, but they are grown for different purposes, and each one comes with its *own legal status*.

The medical marijuana plants are grown to be high in CBD, and they have varying amounts of THC. The CBD oil derived from these plants is regulated by the same state laws governing the use of medical marijuana, and is sold only in MMJ dispensaries.

The FDA considers hemp oil (and its derivative CBD) that comes from industrial hemp plants to be a dietary supplement (not a medication). Therefore, if you live in the U.S., this means you don't need a prescription and can legally purchase and consume CBD from hemp in any state. This CBD oil also has the added benefit of having virtually no THC (less than 1 percent). You cannot get high with CBD hemp oil, and these products can be purchased at several sites on the Internet or in some retail stores. They work quite well for treating anxiety and seizures, less so for sleep disorders, but are not as effective for relieving pain as those derived from marijuana, which has greater amounts of THC.

On December 14, 2016, the Drug Enforcement Administration (DEA) added a notice to the *Federal Register* that quietly informed the public it had established "a new drug code for marihuana extract." The DEA's argument was that the agency was entitled to regulate CBD oil because all extracts contain trace amounts of THC, the active ingredient in cannabis, which remains illegal at the federal level.

Establishing this new drug code is, effectively, the first step toward classifying CBD oil alongside cannabis under the Controlled Substances Act. This act classifies cannabis as a Schedule 1 substance, alongside drugs like heroin that are addictive and considered to have no practical medical benefit.

However, legal experts and advocates for hemp doubt that the DEA has the mandate to easily reclassify CBD oil. But if they are somehow successful in classifying CBD as a Schedule 1 drug, which I doubt they will be, then a pure CBD product (tincture, topical, or oil) could only be legally obtained from a medical marijuana dispensary.

By placing CBD in the same category as heroin makes no rational sense. I hope ongoing research and attention to existing data help to remove CBD (and marijuana) from any consideration as a Schedule 1 drug.

14. Are there other cannabinoids besides CBD and THC that can help relieve pain and reduce inflammation?

Yes, there are several others that have been isolated and are available in some dispensaries:

- THCa—Tetrahydrocannabinolic acid is not only a tongue-twister but also the acidic precursor to THC. In the live cannabis plant, THCa is the most abundant cannabinoid, while THC is present in only minute quantities. After cannabis is harvested, THCa begins to naturally convert to THC. It also converts to THC when burned, vaporized, or heated for a period of time at a specific temperature.

  THCa is not psychoactive, and it appears to be the most potent *anti-inflammatory* of all the cannabinoids. It also inhibits cancer cell growth, reduces muscle spasms, and enhances sleep. THCa interacts with the endocannabinoid system, but not with the CB1 receptors (in the brain).

  Patients often prefer THCa to CBD or THC for long-term use, since it's not psychoactive and it's more therapeutic for reducing inflammation. It has been isolated and can be administered by itself via a tincture (preferred) or transdermal patch or with other cannabinoids by juicing. I discuss each of these delivery methods in the following chapter.

- CBN—Cannabinol is primarily a decomposition product, and is produced when THC is exposed to heat or light. It can also be found in old dry marijuana leaves that have been stored for years. Very little CBN can be found in live cannabis. It is mildly psychoactive, with approximately 10 percent the psychoactivity of THC.

  CBN is an excellent *analgesic, anti-inflammatory*, and *sleep enhancer*; it also reduces muscle spasms and can help glaucoma. At the present time, it can only be administered alone, via capsules or a transdermal patch. But when your marijuana is smoked or vaporized, you are most likely inhaling some CBN along with THC and many other cannabinoids.

- CBC—Cannabichromene is not psychoactive. It is an excellent anti-inflammatory, which therefore makes it a good analgesic. Many patients have experienced considerable pain relief from applying a topical CBC salve to the skin covering their painful joint, back, neck, or shoulder. Other than the topical, CBC cannot be administered as a single isolated cannabinoid. However, most medical marijuana products do contain small amounts of CBC.

- CBG—Cannabigerol is not psychoactive and is commonly found in large quantities in hemp fiber. It is known to be an effective anti-inflammatory, as well as an anticancer and blood pressure–lowering agent, a bone stimulant, and an antibacterial. Recent research indicates that it may eventually prove to be even more medicinal than CBD. There are currently very few MMJ products with high-CBG content. I know of only one indica strain, a 70:30/I:S, Permafrost, that fits this description.

- CBDa—Cannabidiolic acid is the acid, or precursor, form of CBD. It is a strong anti-inflammatory, antiemetic (relieves nausea and vomiting), antibacterial, and anti-proliferative (prevents the spread of cancer cells). Similar to THC, CBD, and THCa, CBDa helps to reprogram cancer cells, causing them to shrink in size.

  The best way to administer CBDa is ingesting raw cannabis flowers and leaves through juicing, since it is only prevalent in cannabis that has *not* been heated (e.g., smoked or vaporized). However, once heat has been applied and it is converted to CBD, it still provides all of the therapeutic benefits conveyed by CBD.

15. What are the most common terpenes?

- Myrcene
  Aroma: Musky, cloves, earthy, herbal with notes of citrus and tropical fruit (it's in the same family as turpentine).
  Therapeutic effects and benefits: Pain relief, anti-inflammatory, antidepressant, relieves muscle tension, aids in sleeplessness, antioxidant, anticarcinogenic, sedating "couch-lock" effect, relaxing
  Also found in: Mango, lemongrass, thyme, hops
  * *High-myrcene cannabis strains*: Pure Kush, El Nino, Himalayan Gold, Skunk #1 (all are indica strains)

- Caryophyllene
  Aroma: Pepper, spicy, woody, cloves
  Therapeutic effects and benefits: Anti-inflammatory (especially good for arthritis), aid in autoimmune disorders, relieves ulcers, gastro-protective

Also found in: Black pepper, cloves, cotton
* *High-caryophyllene cannabis strains*: Hash plant

- Limonene
  Aroma: Citrus
  Therapeutic effects and benefits: Elevated mood, stress relief, antidepressant, antifungal, antibacterial, anticarcinogenic, dissolves gallstones, may treat gastrointestinal problems such as heartburn
  Also found in: Peppermint, fruit rinds, rosemary, juniper
  * *High-limonene cannabis strains*: OG Kush, Super Lemon Haze, Jack the Ripper, Lemon Skunk

- Linalool
  Aroma: Floral, citrus, candy
  Therapeutic effects and benefits: Antianxiety, antidepressant, anticonvulsant, anti-acne, sedation
  Also found in: Lavender
  * *High-linalool cannabis strains*: G-13, Amnesia Haze, Lavender, LA Confidential

- Alpha-Pinene, Beta-Pinene
  Aroma: Pine
  Therapeutic effects and benefits: Alertness, asthma relief, antiseptic, memory retention, counteracts some THC psychoactive effects
  Also found in: Pine needles, rosemary, basil, parsley, dill
  * *High-pinene cannabis strains*: Jack Herer, Chemdawg, Bubba Kush, Trainwreck, Super Silver Haze

  *Not every batch of any given strain will have high levels of these terpenes, as they are subjected to variable growing conditions. The only way to be sure is through a lab's terpene analysis.

16. Why is the discovery of the endocannabinoid system so important?

The strongest evidence supporting the use of cannabis as medicine is that it reduces chronic pain. Both in Colorado and California, more than 90 percent of medical marijuana patients are suffering with chronic pain. But due to marijuana's illegality it has taken the scientific community many years to overcome its resistance to doing the research and beginning to unravel the mystery of what the plant consists of and how it works (if used appropriately) to relieve pain; reduce inflammation, anxiety, and seizures; stimulate appetite; relax muscles; kill cancer cells; and enhance sleep and feelings of well-being.

Dr. Raphael Mechoulam, an Israeli organic chemist, considered the "father of cannabis science," has spent a lifetime studying cannabis. It struck him as odd that even though morphine had been extracted from opium in 1805 and cocaine from coca leaves in 1855, scientists had no idea what the principal psychoactive ingredient was in marijuana. In 1964 he and his research team discovered the highly psychoactive *THC*, and later also elucidated the chemical structure of *CBD*, currently considered the most medicinal cannabinoid.

In 1992 Dr. Mechoulam's ongoing research led him from the cannabis plant itself to the inner recesses of the human brain. That year he and several colleagues made an extraordinary discovery. They isolated the chemical *made by the human body* that binds to the same receptor in the brain that THC does. Mechoulam named it *anandamide*, from the Sanskrit for *"supreme joy,"* and referred to it as an *endocannabinoid*—i.e., originating from inside the body.

Since then there have been more than twenty-one thousand studies and articles that have appeared in scientific publications in the U.S., an average of more than two per day, on the subject of either cannabis or cannabinoids (but relatively few focused on cannabis and pain relief). Not only has this scientific investigation documented a great many healing benefits, but it has also uncovered several other endocannabinoids (a total of five have been identified) and their receptors (CB1 and CB2) comprising the endocannabinoid *system*.

Many of these researchers have concluded that this previously unknown physiologic system (*physiology* = the branch of biology that deals with the normal functions of living organisms and their parts) is a *key component to establishing and maintaining human health*.

Scientists now recognize that endocannabinoids interact with a specific neurological network—much the way that endorphins, serotonin, and dopamine do. In fact, exercise has been shown to elevate endocannabinoid levels in the brain. In an October 2015 study in Germany, researchers concluded that although exercise raises the blood levels of both endorphins and endocannabinoids, it is the *endocannabinoids that are solely responsible for runner's high* (previously thought to result from the endorphins), and they also significantly contribute to the analgesic effect of endorphins (the body's natural opiates).

I found this to be the case whenever I went for a hike during the peak of my bout with shingles. Pain reduction was both dramatic and consistent even without the use of medical marijuana. It worked every time, typically occurred within the first ten to fifteen minutes, and was maintained throughout the duration of the hike. Pain reduction was even greater when I did use marijuana during exercise. But I reserved this use for less strenuous exercise, since it can increase heart rate.

Fueled by the added anecdotal and clinical study reports of potential benefit, advances in understanding of the endocannabinoid signaling system upon which cannabis acts, as well as growing public acceptance that cannabis should be available as a medicine if a physician recommends it, a number of compelling studies have been published in recent years.

Research has revealed that the endocannabinoids are chemically very similar to the cannabinoids found in cannabis, and bind to the same receptors. The mechanism initiating the specific function of each cannabinoid (whether it originates within the body or from cannabis) occurs as it attaches to an endocannabinoid receptor, comparable to a key being inserted into a lock.

These receptors are found throughout the body: in the brain (primarily the CB1 receptors that interact chiefly with THC), organs, connective tissue, glands, and immune cells. CB2 receptors are predominantly found in the immune system and appear to be responsible for analgesic, anti-inflammatory, and other therapeutic effects of cannabis.

In each tissue, the endocannabinoid system performs different tasks, but the goal is always a *steady-state* or *homeostasis* (defined as the maintenance of a stable internal environment despite fluctuations in the external environment). Endocannabinoids promote homeostasis at every level of biological life, playing an important role in such basic functions as memory, balance, movement, immune health, and neuroprotection; reducing pain, inflammation, and anxiety; and inducing sleep and killing cancer cells. Reduction in endocannabinoid levels and/or changes in the CB2 receptors have been reported in almost all diseases affecting humans, ranging from cardiovascular, gastrointestinal, liver, kidney, neurodegenerative, psychiatric, bone, skin, autoimmune, and lung disorders to chronic pain and cancer.

Endocannabinoids are also found at the intersection of the body's various systems—e.g., nervous, digestive, cardiovascular—allowing communication and coordination between different cell types. At the site of an injury, for example, cannabinoids can be found decreasing the release of activators and sensitizers from the injured tissue, stabilizing the nerve cells to prevent excessive firing, and calming nearby immune cells to prevent release of pro-inflammatory substances. Three different mechanisms of action on three different cell types form a single purpose: *minimize the pain and damage caused by the injury.*

The endocannabinoid system, with its complex actions in our immune system, nervous system, and all of the body's organs, is literally a *bridge between body and mind.* By understanding this system we begin to see a mechanism that explains how states of consciousness can promote health or disease by bringing us into a state of balance and harmony. Other than hormones and the endocrine system, there is nothing else in the human body comparable to the multifaceted endocannabinoid system.

As a former biology major in college, with a fascination for the miraculous organism of the human body my entire adult life, I find this information to be quite remarkable. It strongly indicates that *endocannabinoids are vital to the optimal functioning of the human body.*

17. How can marijuana aid end-of-life care?

Marijuana can be extremely helpful for people in hospice care or at home with a terminal condition. It can relieve pain, decrease nausea and vomiting, improve appetite, and help increase energy. Depending upon what therapeutic effect is most needed, the primary caretaker will determine which MMJ product to administer.

For easing pain and increasing energy I suggest using the 1:1/CBD:THC patch. For agitation and mild-moderate pain, you can try the CBD patch (no THC) along with the THCa patch for reducing inflammation (they can be used together). If sleep is a problem and there is pain as well, I would choose the CBN patch. (I discuss this method of administration in the following chapter.) Neither CBD, THCa, nor CBN are psychoactive. Different restrictions apply to the use of MMJ by hospice personnel in each of the twenty-eight states in which it is legal. If hospice is not permitted to administer it, then I would consider doing it yourself if you're comfortable doing so, and if you are the primary caretaker.

Chapter 4

Choosing Your Delivery Method

We're all unique, with our own needs, desires, and body chemistry. There is no one size fits all when it comes to using medical marijuana for treating chronic pain. Each of us will respond somewhat differently to the variety of available products and methods for consuming MMJ. In this chapter I'm presenting you with a multitude of options along with their advantages and disadvantages. From this information you should be able to choose at least one or two methods with which to begin the process of relieving your pain. If you're not satisfied, then try another until you are comfortable with the one you've chosen.

Whatever option you choose, remember to rotate the strain of marijuana you're using (if vaporizing or smoking) or the MMJ product, and to not use the same one every day. It's most effective to have three or four different strains or products available, and don't use the same one for more than three consecutive days. Otherwise you might develop some degree of tolerance, and it will be less effective for pain relief.

SMOKING

Smoking marijuana gained popularity with Americans shortly after the Mexican revolution in the 1920s, with the influx of Mexicans who did it recreationally to relax. Due largely to its convenience and rapid onset, *smoking remains the most popular method of administration.*

Although smoking is by far the most frequently used method, it is certainly not the healthiest way to use marijuana. Smoke is a major irritant to the sensitive mucous membrane lining the entire respiratory tract—nose, sinuses, and lungs. Chronic irritation can lead to inflammation, which in turn causes swelling and a narrowing of the airway. As a result less oxygen is obtained with each breath, and oxygen is our most critical nutrient for optimal health.

Coughing is an immediate response to the irritation from the smoke. However, if you are someone who has preexisting chronic inflammation of the mucous membrane, such as chronic sinusitis, allergies, asthma, or chronic bronchitis, smoking will to some extent increase the inflammation, which in turn can cause increased congestion (nasal, head, or lung), postnasal mucus drainage, cough, possible allergy symptoms, fatigue, and irritability, along with greater susceptibility to infection. In those people with a predisposition to sinus or allergy problems, this increased inflammation can also precipitate a sinus infection or an allergy attack. I found this to be the case during the late 1970s when I would often develop a sinus infection within twenty-four to forty-eight hours following my weekly Sabbath ritual of smoking marijuana.

From early childhood my radiologist father had made me acutely aware of the health risks of smoking cigarettes. He would bring home chest X-rays of patients he had diagnosed earlier that day with lung cancer, and after dinner he would set his view box on the kitchen table, put up the X-ray, and point out the lung tumor. I remember asking him, "Why did this person get lung cancer?" And his response was always the same: "He was a smoker." This was in the mid-1950s, nearly ten years before the surgeon general required a health risk warning on all cigarette box labels in 1964.

Then I'd ask, "What will happen to him?" "He'll die. There's nothing we can do for him" was my father's grave response. He seemed not only truly forlorn for the terminal fate of the patient, but genuinely sad that his beloved medical profession was unable to do anything to help save him. His message to me was conveyed loudly and clearly: "Smoking is a really bad thing to do." During the past sixty years, other than smoking marijuana, I've strictly adhered to his advice.

Until my sinus problems began around the age of thirty, I thought smoking marijuana once or twice a week was relatively harmless. It was a revelation to me that smoke even at this frequency can increase inflammation enough to cause sinus infections. This is especially true when there are other contributing factors present, such as stress, a weakened immune system, or exposure to cold viruses.

The air most Americans are breathing, both outdoor and indoor, is already polluted. We don't need to add another pollutant by smoking anything, whether it is a cigarette or a joint.

Although it was not well known in the 1950s and early '60s, today most Americans are well aware that tobacco smoke contains carcinogens that can cause lung cancer. But surprisingly, several major population studies have shown *no link between marijuana smoking and a higher risk of lung cancer*. In fact, a Jamaican study showed that regular users of marijuana had a lower risk of cancer than nonsmokers!

Both cigarette and marijuana smoke contain carcinogens, but the anticancer properties of several of the cannabinoids, especially THC and CBD, prevent the promotion of lung cancer. To lend greater clarity to this important subject, research has shown that nicotine, the active and highly addictive ingredient in tobacco, activates an enzyme that converts certain chemicals in tobacco smoke into a cancer-promoting form. Conversely, THC inhibits this enzyme from activating the carcinogens found in marijuana smoke.

However, this does not mean that smoking marijuana is risk-free, especially for people suffering with chronic pain, or for current or former sinus, asthma, or allergy sufferers. In the vast majority of cases of chronic pain, there is some degree of underlying inflammation. Smoke contains toxins created from combustion, and when they are inhaled and enter your bloodstream, they can potentially increase inflammation in any part of the body where inflammation already exists (e.g., arthritic knees or hips). This is in addition to the increased inflammation resulting from direct contact of the smoke and heated air on the mucous membrane lining the respiratory tract. Several of the cannabinoids have an anti-inflammatory effect and can diminish this response, which is another reason marijuana is healthier smoke than tobacco, but it's still smoke. And with smoke there are risks that can and should be avoided by chronic pain patients, especially those suffering with migraine headaches. Smoke is a potential *trigger* for migraine.

Another potential risk from smoking marijuana is respiratory infections, such as sinusitis, bronchitis, and pneumonia, resulting from contamination with bacteria and fungi. In Colorado, surprisingly after nearly seven years of legalized medical marijuana, *required* microbiology testing for MMJ has not yet been enforced. I have recently heard from a microbiologist who runs a marijuana testing facility that following preliminary laboratory tests performed by the state, it is estimated that as much as 70 percent of the marijuana in Colorado will have tested positive for the aspergillus fungus. (This finding has not been officially confirmed.) In a person with a weakened immune system, this can cause a serious lung condition called aspergillosis. It is not the fungus itself but the spores of aspergillus that cause the damage, and the spores cannot be destroyed by fire.

I have not smoked marijuana in more than five years. Whether it's a joint (marijuana "cigarette"), pipe, bong, or water pipe, there's combustion, and smoke is always a by-product. Given the potential health risks, and as a former sinus sufferer, I prefer a much safer alternative for inhaling the flower and obtaining an immediate effect . . . *vaporizers*.

Advantages of smoking: Immediate and possibly stronger effect (for some people) than with a vaporizer; allows user to choose most effective strain from among a wide variety of strains of flower; for veteran "pot smokers" the aroma (conveyed by terpenes) is more evident.

Disadvantages of smoking: Most unhealthy method of administration (causes inflammation and greater susceptibility to infection), especially to the respiratory tract; smoke produces an odor that may be offensive to others and makes it more difficult to be discreet while using. Smoking provides the shortest duration of action—two to three hours.

VAPORIZING

Vaporizers are essentially miniature "ovens" that heat but do not burn the marijuana, at temperatures ranging from 360 to 420 degrees Fahrenheit. There is no flame, and no combustion, and therefore none of the toxins that accompany marijuana smoke. This allows the user to inhale only the psychoactive and medicinal cannabinoids within the specific strain being vaporized.

There is a vast difference in the quality of "smoke" that one receives when marijuana is vaporized versus when it is smoked. Approximately 88 percent of the combusted smoke gases contain non-cannabinoid elements, most of which provide potential health risks. Conversely when one uses a vaporizer, the smoke (actually a thick vapor) and gases that are inhaled consist of approximately 95 percent cannabinoids, which are largely medicinal.

Vaporizers can be purchased in a wide variety of shapes, sizes, and prices. Although most vaporizers that accommodate only the marijuana flower are in the $200 to $500 range, the one I personally use and recommend to patients, the Fully Alive Vaporizer® (formerly the Wulf-LX), sells for $95 (see Resources). The Volcano has for several years been regarded as the "gold standard" of vaporizers, and it retails for more than $500. Having used one on three different occasions, I consider it the best example of effective marketing I've ever seen. It's simply not worth it. And since expense is a deterrent to using a vaporizer for many medical marijuana patients, I would like to make it clear that it is *not* necessary to exceed $100 to purchase an excellent vaporizer.

Even though to veteran "pot smokers" the effect derived from vaporizing may not be quite the same (many tell me without specifics, "I don't like it as much," while others have said, "It doesn't smell the same"), I can assure you that for inhaling the medical marijuana flower and obtaining an *immediate medicinal effect*, vaporizers work quite well. In fact, *inhalation (smoking or vaporizing) is the* only *method of administration that conveys almost immediate pain relief.*

It does help when using a vaporizer to keep in mind these guidelines:

- The optimum temperature for vaporization is 375 degrees—at this temperature there is little or no visible "smoke" (it's actually a thick vapor); a good quality vaporizer allows you to set the exact temperature. If you find 375 degrees to be too harsh, I'd suggest a setting of 360 degrees, but you may need to take additional inhalations at this temperature to obtain the desired effect.
- Use a grinder to break the flower/bud into small pieces (rather than crumbling it with your fingers) before placing them in the vaporizer chamber; preferably a grinder with three levels and a screen separating

the second and third levels to capture the tiny particles of kief. These are the resin glands that contain the cannabinoids and terpenes that make each strain of cannabis unique. Once you've collected a moderate amount of kief at the base of the grinder, these can then be sprinkled into the chamber of the vaporizer along with the flower to obtain an enhanced effect. The use of a grinder enables you to maximize the effect of vaporizing while avoiding wasting any part of the plant.

- For every one hit or inhalation of smoke (if you were previously a smoker), you should do two hits on the vaporizer; four to six inhalations (the equivalent of two to three hits of smoke) is nearly always sufficient to feel the desired effect. If you tend to be someone who is especially sensitive to most drugs, then start with only two or three hits. Your final inhalation can be immediately after you've turned off the vaporizer, since there is still vapor available.
- To make vaporizing more gentle and less irritating to your lungs, do not take an excessively deep breath or hold your breath at the end of each inhalation. Breathe normally and take your breaths in fairly rapid succession. The longer you wait between hits, the more "cooked" the marijuana will be, the thicker the vapor you'll be inhaling, the more visible the vapor that you will exhale, and the more irritating it will be to your lungs.

Most people will notice the medicinal or psychoactive effect within two to five minutes. And with both smoking and vaporizing it will typically last for two to three hours. Although the other methods of administration require more time before you feel the effect, they do last longer than with inhalation. The other benefit is that these methods do no harm to your respiratory tract. For those medical marijuana patients with even mild or moderate chronic inflammation of the respiratory mucous membrane, 375-degree air is still an irritant and can increase inflammation, albeit not nearly to the same extent as smoke. My recommendation to these patients is to avoid using a vaporizer as long as you still have inflammation (you'll know you're inflamed by virtue of your symptoms—nasal congestion, cough, excessive mucus); or set the temperature at 360 degrees, and see how you react.

For those patients with chronic pain and sleep problems (the pain often awakens them), without any inflammation of their respiratory tract, the following vaporizing techniques can be quite helpful:

- Shortly before bed, vaporize at 375 degrees a strain that you've found to be effective for pain and sleep (e.g., a strong indica).
- After you've finished vaporizing do not empty the chamber, but raise the temperature setting to 395 degrees and then turn the vaporizer off.
- Place the vaporizer within reach, on your nightstand by the bed, before going to sleep.
- If after three to four hours you awaken with (or without) pain, you can turn on the vaporizer and take two to four hits at 395 degrees. Even though you are using the same leaves you've previously vaporized at 375 degrees, it will still work quite well for relieving your pain and making you sleepy. This entire process will have taken just a few minutes before you're back to sleep. And since the vaporizer is already loaded, with the temperature at the appropriate setting, there's no need to get up out of bed or even to turn on any lights.

This technique illustrates an additional advantage of using a vaporizer that allows you to set the temperature. You're able to use the same leaves more than once, which is extremely helpful for people who have problems with both falling and staying asleep. You can more easily get a good night's sleep with minimal interruption. Since medical marijuana is not inexpensive, if you're interested in saving money and did not need to use the vaporizer a second time during the night, you can use it the following night without refilling it with fresh leaves. Keep in mind, however, that there is more "smoke" (thicker vapor) at the higher temperatures and a greater likelihood of stimulating a cough. I only recommend this method if you have a healthy respiratory tract. And if so, it's possible to use the same leaves a third time by raising the temperature another 15 to 20 degrees, to somewhere between 410 and 415.

Another money-saving tip for those with healthy respiratory tracts is the possibility of smoking the leaves that have already been vaporized, or even better, you may use them for making edibles.

Advantages of vaporizing: Immediate effect with little or no smoke, odor, or damage to the respiratory tract; allows user to choose most effective strain from among a wide variety of strains of flower, to determine optimum dose (number of inhalations or "hits") for pain relief, to save money by re-vaporizing the same flower more than once (only with a healthy respiratory tract), and to use the vaporized leaves to make edibles; with no smoke or odor the user can be more discreet.

Disadvantages of vaporizing: Can be somewhat irritating to those with preexisting inflammation of respiratory tract; weaker aroma and terpene effect. Vaporizers that accommodate *only oil cartridges* greatly limit your choice of specific strains. Duration of action is only two to three hours.

SMOKING OR VAPORIZING IN SPITE OF HAVING RESPIRATORY PROBLEMS

As I've mentioned, smoking is unhealthy for anyone. And if you're a sinus sufferer, have serious nasal allergies, asthma, chronic cough, or any other respiratory problem, it is best to avoid vaporizing as well. However, I do understand the difficulty of stopping an enjoyable habit, even though there are a number of other healthier options for using marijuana.

As I explained in the Introduction to this book, very often a health crisis can become a gift. In 1980, I was diagnosed with chronic sinusitis and told I would have to live with it. Although I rejected that prognosis and was determined to cure the condition, I also recognized that I'd have to stop smoking marijuana in order to achieve my goal. This grievous loss of one of my life's greatest pleasures served as a powerful motivator for the development of the holistic *Sinus Survival* program and the writing of a book that quickly became a bestseller.

Prior to 1980, I rarely smoked more than twice a week. But even at that frequency I often developed a sinus infection within a day or two after smoking. If my treatment program worked, then I'd be able to smoke (no more than two or three hits) without getting a sinus infection. This benchmark became a primary measure (although certainly not the only one) of my progress in healing my sinuses.

I stopped smoking entirely for more than a year, and allowed my body to heal the mucous membrane, at least to some extent (living in

Denver, I was still breathing polluted and dry air). At the same time I made other changes with regard to diet and nasal hygiene practices. Through a trial-and-error process I gradually reintroduced smoking back into my life. Smoking marijuana provided an excellent method for both challenging and evaluating the health of my inflamed mucous membrane. As a result it was instrumental in helping to develop a highly effective method for treating and preventing sinus infections, especially in high-risk situations. The method's success, however, was quite limited with smokers of cigarettes (those who smoked at least one half to one pack per day). I finally made the cessation of cigarette smoking a requirement before agreeing to help chronic sinusitis patients implement the holistic medical treatment program.

If you have a respiratory condition, are in the habit of smoking medical marijuana daily or more than once a day to treat your chronic pain, and are unable or unwilling to stop smoking, in spite of the many healthier options presented in this chapter, I suggest utilizing the following components of the Respiratory Healing program to prevent infection and mitigate inflammation whenever you smoke or vaporize:

- *Saline nasal spray*: Preferably one that contains anti-inflammatory and anti-infective herbs, such as the Sinus Survival Nasal Spray (containing aloe and berberis): two sprays in each nostril just before smoking, and again within fifteen to twenty minutes after smoking. This will lessen inflammation and reduce risk of infection, while cleansing and moistening the mucous membrane. The most effective way to spray is to tilt your head slightly forward, tilt the head of the spray bottle toward the *outside* of each nostril (not towards the septum dividing your nostrils), and gently inhale as you spray. Sinus Survival products are available online (see Resources).
- *Peppermint oil*: Use immediately following the nasal spray; place a few drops on your index (first) finger, touch this finger to your thumb and then swab (with both finger and thumb) around the *outside* of both nostrils. This will stimulate blood flow to your mucous membrane, increase absorption of the medicinal herbs that you just sprayed, and act as a decongestant. Available at health food stores or as Sinus Essentials oil online (see Resources).

- *Steam inhaler*: This may be the single most effective method for protecting your mucous membrane. It should be used shortly (within twenty to thirty minutes) after you've smoked. Add filtered water to the cup at the base of the steamer, and after it begins steaming, add two to three sprays of a highly medicinal eucalyptus oil, for example Sinus Survival Eucalyptus. (Eucalyptus oil acts as a potent anti-inflammatory, but less than 2 percent of the approximately seven hundred species of eucalyptus are truly medicinal.) Then add a few drops of peppermint oil and tea tree oil to the steam. Sit with your nose and mouth close to or touching the plastic hood of the steamer for at least fifteen to twenty minutes. Be aware that the eucalyptus oil might initially stimulate a cough, but that will rarely last for more than a few seconds. Studies have shown steaming to reduce inflammation and nasal congestion, an ideal balance to smoking, which increases both. Tea tree oil can help to kill viruses, bacteria, and fungi. Steam inhalers are available at most pharmacies; and Sinus Survival Eucalyptus, Tea Tree, and Peppermint oils for steam therapy are available online (see Resources).

- *Nasal irrigation*: For those with chronic sinusitis, it is very helpful to irrigate your nose and sinuses immediately following the steaming. The most effective irrigating device is a pulsatile irrigator called SinuPulse, which utilizes the same technology as the Waterpik device for teeth. Studies have shown pulsatile irrigators to be the only devices capable of removing biofilm, a thick coating of mucus typically found on the surface of a chronically inflamed mucous membrane. SinuPulse can be purchased online (see Resources) and other irrigators are available at most pharmacies.

- *Diet*: Avoid inflammatory (acidic) foods, especially milk and dairy products, alcohol, caffeine, and sugar (see Acid/Alkaline Food Chart in Chapter 5). Be conscious of drinking lots of water after smoking or vaporizing, to counter the dryness of the mucous membrane triggered by marijuana, as mentioned previously in Chapter 3 (question 8 "side effects of THC").

- *Anger*: Avoid smoking marijuana if you're angry. The emotion of anger, especially if it's repressed, can significantly increase inflammation.

- *Don't hold your breath*: Breathe normally to avoid prolonged exposure of the mucous membrane to smoke and heated air.

- *Purchase only marijuana that you know has undergone microbiology testing*: This will help to avoid bacterial (e.g., staph) and fungal (e.g., aspergillosis) infections.

Even though these suggestions will all help to significantly mitigate inflammation and help prevent infection of the respiratory tract, they cannot completely eliminate the negative effects of smoking. You will do a much better job of self-care if you choose one or more of the following methods of administration while you're healing your respiratory tract.

TINCTURES

Tinctures are one of many forms of marijuana concentrate. However, I will cover them separately in this section, because they deserve more attention, and the other commonly used concentrates in the following section.

In the very near future, I expect to see cannabis *tinctures and other forms of trans-mucosal delivery systems*—including intra-nasal and sublingual (under tongue) sprays and drops in addition to sublingual and oral (dissolve in mouth) tablets—*become the preferred and most recommended method* (by physicians) *for administering medical marijuana.* Scientific and technological advances in the modern age will provide us with the most potent pain-relieving cannabis tinctures and other trans-mucosal delivery methods ever produced. The majority of doctors and their medical marijuana patients will rely on tinctures (and the soon-to-be-released trans-mucosal products) to provide rapid onset of action; improved dosing, safety, and effectiveness; and a convenient means of administration.

Tinctures are not new. The fact that cannabis was administered as a tincture in several of the most popular medicines for nearly a century (beginning in the mid-1800s) has been largely forgotten. Until cannabis was declared illegal in 1937, *tinctures were the only type of cannabis medicines in the U.S.* The word *marijuana* and the practice of smoking the cannabis plant came to America from Mexico. It was brought here by the thousands of immigrants who arrived in the U.S. during and following the Mexican revolution (1910–1920). Americans were not familiar with the word *marijuana* or the practice of smoking the plant, but they were well aware that cannabis was the key ingredient in many of their most popular medicines, especially those used for treating arthritis, migraine, menstrual pain, neuralgia (nerve pain), and depression.

Tinctures are liquid concentrates typically produced via alcohol extraction. They are extractions of *whole plant* cannabis (usually produced from the flowers and trim leaves), containing all of the cannabinoids and terpenes in the specific strain from which they were extracted. They are relatively easy to make and inexpensive.

Tinctures are absorbed both sublingually and through the oral mucosa (tissue lining the mouth). Titration or dose control is easily achieved by the number of drops patients place under their tongue, where the medicine is rapidly absorbed into tiny blood vessels and quickly transported to the brain and body. A minimum of two to three minutes of holding the tincture under the tongue is generally recommended. That will work, but I've found that for more complete and faster absorption and a subsequent stronger peak effect, it's helpful to keep the tincture in your mouth (sloshing it around and letting it sit under and surrounding your tongue) for a much longer time frame. I've found that ten to fifteen minutes is optimum. When the tincture is held for that length of time, the psychoactive effect can sometimes begin within twenty to twenty-five minutes of inserting the drops.

Rapidity of onset is especially important to those patients suffering with migraine headaches. As you'll learn in Chapter 8, although MMJ is highly effective for preventing and relieving a migraine headache, in order for it to do its job, it has to take effect within the brief window between the aura (early warning) and full-blown headache.

It will often take between thirty and forty-five minutes before patients begin to notice the effects of an MMJ tincture, and an additional forty-five to sixty minutes before they reach their peak. This maximum effect can then last for another four to five hours. It takes less time to begin feeling it, and the maximum effect is stronger and lasts longer, if you have an empty stomach and/or engage in moderate exercise (for at least twenty to thirty minutes) preceding its administration. Total duration of the medicinal effect of tinctures is four to six hours.

If after ninety minutes patients are not experiencing the desired effect, I instruct them to add more drops, and wait to see how the stronger dose is working. This method of individualizing the dosage (called *self-titration*) clearly distinguishes cannabis tinctures from pharmaceutical drugs, which are most often prescribed in a one-size-fits-all fashion. The opportunity for patients to easily determine the optimal dose for their unique body and their specific condition makes tinctures the *ideal self-care medicine*.

Tinctures can be flavored for better taste. They are best stored in dark bottles in the refrigerator. Since tinctures average about 75 percent ethanol, there is little worry of bacterial or other biological contamination. For those who wish to avoid alcohol, a California company, Yolo Botanicals, sells Prana Bio Medicinals, providing patients with alcohol-free, sugar-free tinctures. Prana Bio Medicinal products are formulated from a variety of pure plant CBD-rich and THC-based cannabis strains with specific ratios and terpene profiles, divided into categories called P1 (THC:THCa), P2 (3:1 CBD), P3 (1:1 CBD), P4 (CBD:CBN), P5 (CBD:CBDa), available in capsule, sublingual, and topical delivery methods. P1 thru P3 are available in activated (with THC) or non-activated (without THC) formulas, offering patients options between a psychoactive or non-psychoactive therapy. Prana's unique tinctures are infused in pharmaceutical-grade fatty acids. This not only eliminates the need for alcohol or ethanol, but greatly increases their bioavailability. Since marijuana is fat-soluble, the rate of absorption for these tinctures is far superior to that for others.

I was most impressed with the analgesic and sleep-inducing effect P4 had on my shingles pain. However, it became unavailable in Colorado and I was unable to continue using it.

I believe we will soon see a rapid development of cannabis tinctures, as the weaknesses of the other methods of administration become more apparent. I'm excited about the wide of variety of *trans-mucosal delivery systems* that will soon be available, in addition to the sublingual drops and sprays currently available. There will also be more tinctures not using alcohol as their extraction method. Current tinctures include:

- Indica, sativa, and hybrid
- 1:1, 2:1, 3:1, 6:1, 20:1/CBD:THC—Each of these tinctures is excellent for relieving pain, and the 20:1 is best for sleep and pain, with a minimal psychoactive effect. (A Boulder-based company, marQaha, recently created a new tincture made from the Harlequin strain with CBD:THC of 1:1. I believe it is currently the strongest analgesic of all tinctures, besides producing a pleasant high.)
- THCa—Not psychoactive, and possibly the *most potent anti-inflammatory* of all cannabinoids. It closely parallels the effect of THCa obtained from juicing raw cannabis leaves, which makes this tincture the most practical and therapeutic method for obtaining THCa. It's more effective than the transdermal patch, and raw cannabis leaves are not readily available. Since it's not psychoactive, it can be used *in conjunction with any of the other tinctures or other methods of MMJ administration*. This combination can offer great relief for patients suffering with highly inflammatory conditions such as rheumatoid arthritis or Crohn's disease.
- CBD/CBN with low THC—These are ideal for reducing pain and promoting sleep.
- CBD tinctures—From either hemp or marijuana, they are not psychoactive and the latest research reveals these to be most effective for reducing anxiety and some seizures, and moderately (at best) helpful for relieving pain or enhancing sleep. I'm familiar with an excellent CBD hemp oil (no THC) combined with phospholipids (liposomes = healthy fats), available through Quicksilver Scientific in Lafayette, Colorado.

Advantages of tinctures: Most convenient, safest, and most consistently reliable method for determining optimal dose, referred to as self-titrating. They have a longer duration of action than smoking or vaporizing. Tinctures are the most conducive method for creating unique formulas and combinations of individual cannabinoids, especially CBD, THCa, CBN, and THC. Of the non-inhalation methods, tinctures are among the most consistent or homogenized dosed formulas—i.e., they are more uniform throughout. This means that each drop of the tincture has approximately the same amount of CBD, THC, or any of the other cannabinoids as every other drop. The lack of homogeneity is a significant problem with edibles. It is not surprising that a century ago, tinctures were the *only* method of administering cannabis medicine.

Disadvantages of tinctures: Limited selection, with most medical dispensaries having relatively few choices of tinctures for sale. Most tinctures contain alcohol.

CONCENTRATES OR EXTRACTS (OTHER THAN TINCTURES)

Cannabis concentrates include any cannabis product produced through an extraction process. Solvents such as butane, CO_2, and ethanol strip compounds from the cannabis plant, leaving behind a product with cannabinoids packed in every drop. Some types of extracts, such as shatter and wax, test as high as 90 to 95 percent THC (three to four times higher than the strongest sativa strains of flower), while others are rich in non-psychoactive compounds, most often CBD. But it is the extremely high THC content that makes these concentrates such a potent and *high-risk* medicine. Although they are classified as concentrates, tinctures as whole-plant extracts do not have nearly as high a concentration of THC as shatter and wax. These stronger concentrates are typically consumed through dabbing (see below) and vaporizing.

There is also a significant safety issue with the production of extracts, but this can be minimized with the use of a professional extractor and other more sophisticated equipment. Butane is highly flammable and mildly toxic. Before purchasing, check to confirm that the butane hash oil (BHO) is lab tested for purity, as improperly purged BHO may contain traces of butane, which should be avoided. The other extraction methods, such as CO_2 or ice-water extraction, are much healthier and safer, and reduce or remove the possibility of explosions.

Hash

The oldest and most familiar form of concentrate is hash or hashish, a cannabis product made by compression of the plant's resin. The powdery kief that coats the cannabis flowers can be collected (as described above with a grinder in the "Vaporizing" section) and pressed together to form hash, or solvents like ice water or ethanol may be used to more effectively strip the plant of its cannabinoid-loaded crystals. Though not as popular or as potent (nor does it have the potential risk of rendering the endocannabinoid receptors ineffective) as the other cannabis concentrates, hashish remains a staple of cannabis culture around the world. It is typically smoked, and is not conducive to vaporizing.

CO_2 or Butane Hash Oil (BHO)

Butane hash oil (BHO) is a high-potency concentrate that has been extracted from the plant using the chemical butane. Butane is convenient and widely available, making it ideal for this process. However, butane is also a mildly toxic chemical (found as well in common scent and flavor extracts), highly flammable, and can be dangerous to work with. For these reasons, many dispensaries are switching to CO_2 as the preferred method of extraction. It is healthier to inhale or ingest and safer to work with.

Hash oils are available as sativa, indica, and hybrid; as well as in a variety of CBD:THC ratios. BHO or CO_2 hash oil is a thick, dark brown, sticky substance most often dispensed in a syringe. The recommended dose is an amount approximately the size of one grain of rice. (Start with less if you are someone who is particularly sensitive to drugs.) It can either be vaporized (only with vaporizers that can accommodate oil) or ingested. I recommend the latter since its duration of action is more than twice as long (six to eight hours) as vaporizing (two to three hours). In addition, vaporizing the oil requires a much higher temperature than the flower (440 degrees Fahrenheit versus 375 degrees) and is therefore more harsh on the mucous membrane lining the respiratory tract.

I suggest eating it with a fatty food—e.g., avocado or peanut butter—since marijuana is fat-soluble and this will allow for more rapid absorption, sometimes as quickly as thirty to forty-five minutes. Otherwise it might take one to even two hours to feel a strong therapeutic effect. Since the oil is so sticky, it helps to push it out of the syringe onto a relatively hard surface, such as a cracker, and then you can scrape off the remaining oil at the opening of the syringe onto the cracker. After the dose of oil has been dispensed, then add your fatty food, and eat all of it. I don't recommend eating a sizable meal along with the oil, unless it's an especially fatty meal. A big meal will significantly delay the onset of the hash oil.

Rick Simpson Oil (RSO)

In 2003 a man named Rick Simpson treated his skin cancer using a homemade remedy made from cannabis. When he soaked the cannabis in pure naphtha or isopropyl alcohol, the therapeutic compounds were drawn out of the plant, leaving behind a tar-like liquid after the solvent fully evaporated. Also known as *Phoenix Tears,* Rick Simpson Oil (RSO) can be orally administered or applied directly to the skin. There are several dispensaries currently selling their own versions of the oil, some of which are high in THC while others contain only minimal amounts, along with a relatively high percentage of CBD.

Since THC and CBD both have anticancer properties, the most effective oil for treating cancer combines the two, with significant amounts of both. RSO is considered to be the most effective MMJ product for treating cancer, both ingested and applied topically to skin cancers. (This treatment should be used as a complement to conventional cancer treatment.) The most frequent complaint expressed by patients ingesting RSO is that "it makes me too high." I recently heard from a patient who has been administering the RSO in rectal suppositories (he fills the capsules himself from the syringe he purchases at the dispensary), and the psychoactive effect is greatly diminished.

Although RSO can be produced in a variety of ways, it is traditionally done with an alcohol extract. Dispensing and dosing are similar to what I've described for CO_2 hash oil above.

Shatter and Wax

These concentrates are derived from and considered a subcategory of hash oil. The primary differences between hash oil, shatter, and wax are the *consistency* of the end product following the extraction process and the *concentration* of THC. Shatter and wax can have a far greater THC content than hash oil, with as much as 95 percent (or more).

Shatter, with its flawless amber transparency, has a glass-like appearance. Heat, moisture, and high terpene content can affect the texture of the hash oil, turning it into a runnier substance that resembles sap (hence the commonly used nickname *sap*). Oil with a consistency that falls somewhere between glassy shatter and viscous sap, is often referred to as *pull-and-snap*.

The name *cannabis wax* refers to the softer, opaque oils that have lost their transparency after extraction. Unlike those of transparent oils, the molecules of cannabis wax crystallize as a result of agitation. Light can't travel through irregular molecular densities, thus leaving a solid non-transparent oil as the end result.

Just as transparent oils span the spectrum between shatter and sap, wax can also take on different consistencies based on heat, moisture, and the texture of the oil before it is purged (the process in which residual solvents are removed from the product). Runny oils with more moisture tend to form gooey waxes often called *budder*, while the harder ones are likely to take on a soft, brittle texture known as *crumble* or *honeycomb*. The term *wax* can be used to describe all of these softer or solid textures.

Both shatter and wax are typically inhaled through the process of *dabbing*. A *dab* refers to a dose of concentrate that is heated on a hot surface, usually a nail, and then inhaled through a *dab rig*. This method of administering shatter and wax makes dabbing the fastest and most efficient way to relieve pain, and to also get very high. This fact has triggered valid concerns regarding dabbing and the use of shatter and wax.

I do not recommend the use of shatter or wax, except under the most extreme circumstances—i.e., the most severe pain (8 to 10). Even then, it is not necessary. I suffered with shingles pain at a level from an 8 to a 10 for nearly two months. Vaporizing hybrid and indica flower, taking tinctures, ingesting edibles, and applying transdermal patches were enough to reduce the pain to tolerable levels and allowed me to function reasonably well.

Advantages of concentrates/extracts: The greatest benefit of concentrates is that they provide a powerful dose of medicine to those who truly need it, especially for severe pain and, with Rick Simpson Oil/Phoenix Tears, for treating cancer (in conjunction with conventional medical treatment). The safest way to use concentrates is to ingest CO_2-extracted hash oil or RSO. This method also provides the longest-lasting pain relief. Patients dealing with acute severe pain, a flare-up of chronic pain, or extreme nausea report that dabbing can be the most effective way to get immediate relief. I've also heard from a few patients with migraine headaches that if they are unable to vaporize flower during the initial window between the early warning and the onset of pain, and they're left with intractable disabling pain, dabbing can relieve it. Once a migraine begins, this seems to be the only method of delivering marijuana capable of significantly reducing the pain.

Disadvantages of concentrates/extracts: With increased use of high-potency concentrates such as shatter and wax, we are recognizing previously unknown risks. As a result of their efficiency in relieving pain, there is a great temptation to use these concentrates on a daily basis, and subsequent dependence, abuse, and addiction are often the result. When shatter and wax are consumed daily, at the very least it results in developing a tolerance and a significant reduction in the therapeutic effect. At worst, it can cause the "burnout" or destruction of the endocannabinoid receptors and can render them inoperable. If this occurs, then marijuana delivered by any method of administration *will have no effect*.

I've seen two patients with severe chronic pain have this happen, and it's very sad indeed. They've had to return to using the prescription narcotics they had weaned themselves off months and years earlier through the use of medical marijuana. The good news is that although it might take several months of complete abstinence from all marijuana for the receptor cells to rejuvenate, the body is capable of recovering.

Dabbing, not surprisingly, is most popular with consumers in their twenties. As stated previously, high-THC marijuana products can be damaging to a developing brain. There's nothing higher in THC content than shatter and wax. This fact leads to another liability of dabbing and inhaling these "super-concentrates." They are responsible for *cannabis abuse*, and for the first time it is now possible to *overdose on cannabis*. For this reason, and their potential for addiction, shatter and wax have been referred to as the *crack cocaine of cannabis*. While they are still not lethal, taking too many dabs can lead to extremely uncomfortable highs and, in some cases, passing out. Although they relieve the pain, they often render the user unable to function. Marijuana has been considered an extremely safe medicinal herb, but the overuse of these high-potency concentrates could be undermining this message of safety. In addition, there have also been reports of more intense withdrawal symptoms for dabbers, but that information is still limited.

The concentrates are in need of more research, and rapidly advancing technology in this field will likely (and hopefully) result in less dabbing. While there is great potential for the use of shatter and wax in treating severe pain, at the present time I do not recommend using them. But if that is your choice, I advise using them with utmost caution, and only for the most severe pain.

EDIBLES

Edibles are food infused with cannabis. They can be purchased in a wide variety of shapes and sizes, including cookies, gummies, cakes, hard candies, chocolate bars, and beverages. Depending on the strain(s) of cannabis used to make them, there are sativa, indica, and hybrid edibles, producing effects much like those described in Chapter 3 for each of these three types of marijuana flower. There are also high-CBD/low-THC edibles that are effective for treating anxiety, pain, and insomnia.

Since edibles are absorbed through the gastrointestinal tract, there are a number of variables that can impact their rate and degree of effectiveness. What, when, and the amount you have eaten prior to or along with ingesting an edible will influence its rate of onset. The condition of the tissue lining the bowel, your weight, and your metabolic rate are additional factors affecting absorption. Rich and dense products such as brownies or chocolate also take longer to digest, which means it will take longer for you to feel the effect. On the other hand, infused drinks begin to work much faster.

As previously mentioned, marijuana is fat-soluble and is therefore absorbed more quickly if you eat it with a fatty food. I suggest not eating a big meal, but some food (including fat) is preferred over an empty stomach.

Given all of these variables, the onset of action of an edible can take from forty-five minutes to two hours.

Advantages of edibles: Edibles provide a discreet and convenient way to consume cannabis, particularly for those chronic pain sufferers looking for an alternative to smoking or vaporizing. They are economical, especially if you make your own. This entails a relatively simple process of first making cannabutter (made by heating butter along with marijuana and then straining out the leaves). You will need sufficient plants and the specific strains that you have found to be helpful for relieving your symptoms. You can either purchase these strains from a dispensary or buy the seeds and grow your own plants.

Other than avoiding inhalation, perhaps the greatest benefit of edibles is their *duration of action*. Depending on the dose, the therapeutic effect can last from four to twelve hours, but on average, you can usually count on six to eight hours of relief. In addition to lasting longer, for some patients the effect can also be more intense than with smoking or vaporizing.

In many cases of inflammatory bowel disease, such as Crohn's and colitis, and even with IBS, edibles seem to be the most effective method of administration.

Disadvantages of edibles: Many medical marijuana patients have had unpleasant and uncomfortable experiences with edibles because they "took too much." When this occurs, the advantage of a long duration of action becomes a distinct disadvantage. You might feel heightened anxiety and unable to function for a significant part of a day. Signs of an edible overdose may include paranoia, lack of coordination, and hallucinations. Some have described this experience as similar to having taken a hallucinogen or being on an "acid trip."

If you feel like you've overdosed, don't panic. Remember, the symptoms will subside within a few hours. Stay calm and hydrated and eat food. Those who have suffered through such an experience are unlikely to want to try an edible a second time.

This has been a common problem with edibles (officially described in the cannabis industry as manufactured infused products—MIPs), which can occur as a result of inconsistency of dosage, the lack of homogeneity in the product (cannabinoids are not evenly distributed), and the accompanying unpredictability of their effects and especially of their response time. These overdose incidents typically occur because the consumer isn't feeling any effect in thirty or forty-five minutes, becomes impatient, and decides to ingest more.

In Colorado, recently revised limits on THC content and new regulations regarding packaging and dosing instructions have helped considerably in decreasing the incidence of overdosing with edibles. State laws now require that total milligrams of THC and number of servings be included on packages. In Colorado, one package cannot have more than one hundred milligrams of THC, and one serving can constitute up to ten milligrams of THC. It is easier to discern the amount that constitutes one serving of some edibles than of others.

Each of us will react a bit differently, and your reaction to the same edibles may vary from one time to the next, depending on the previously described variables. If they're using a particular edible for the first time, I strongly advise patients to start slowly, with a relatively small dose (preferably half the recommended dose on the package) and wait at least an hour (or more) to see how they react before taking a bit more.

For the uninformed consumer, ingesting an edible for the first time can pose a problem. Since medical and recreational marijuana have become legal in Colorado, emergency room visits for marijuana overdose have seen a significant increase. Nearly all of these patients, many of whom are young children, have ingested an edible. This illustrates another liability of edibles for medical marijuana patients with toddlers in the house. The edibles must be kept out of reach, and it must be made clear to the child that they are medicine, not candy.

If edibles are used appropriately, each of these liabilities can be mitigated, and for many chronic pain patients edibles can be quite helpful, in spite of being somewhat unpredictable.

TABLETS, CAPSULES, AND SUPPOSITORIES

Tablets and capsules can be regarded as similar to either tinctures, edibles, or concentrates, depending on the specific product. There are *sublingual tablets* that dissolve quickly under the tongue and can be absorbed within a few minutes and begin to take effect within twenty-five to thirty minutes. Similar to tinctures, their duration of action is four to six hours. This delivery method is a recent addition to the rapidly expanding list of MMJ products. The one with which I'm most familiar is the line of MED-a-mints, available in sativa, hybrid, and indica sublingual tablets. They work well (especially the indica for sleep, the hybrid for pain, and the sativa for migraine), are absorbed quickly, and have a pleasant mint flavor. The manufacturer is planning to introduce a line of high-CBD MED-a-mints sometime in 2017 (see Resources).

There are also *tablets that are swallowed*, and as such, similar to an edible. They can take forty-five to sixty minutes to begin working and can last as long as six to eight hours. The line of Stratos tablets is available in sativa (called *Energy*), hybrid (*Relax*), and indica (*Sleep*), as well as two new high-CBD tablets (15:1 and 1:1/CBD:THC). I've seen excellent results with patients who have taken the indica for sleep.

Some dispensaries sell *capsules containing hash oil* as a more consistent and convenient way of delivering (ingesting) and dosing the oil, rather than dispensing it via a syringe. A few dispensaries now sell *CBD oil* (containing no THC) in capsules in strengths of 10, 25, and 50 mg. CBD capsules are also available online (see Resources).

There are also a few dispensaries that have oil-filled rectal and vaginal *suppositories*. The rectal suppositories begin working within ten to fifteen minites, can last from four to eight hours, and, in some cases, will significantly minimize the psychoactive effect. To learn more about the administration of rectal suppositories visit http://phoenixtears.ca /dosage-information/.

Advantages of tablets and capsules: I'm hopeful that the sublingual tablets will provide an effective option for preventing migraine headaches. Other than smoking, vaporizing, and to a lesser extent, topicals, the sativa or hybrid MED-a-mints are the only other current delivery method that can potentially work quickly enough to knock out the headache before a full-blown migraine puts you out of commission. And they are much more convenient than those other methods. However, their effect is dependent on the length of time between the early warning or aura of an imminent migraine and when the pain actually sets in. If this window is less than twenty-five to thirty minutes, it will not be as effective as vaporizing.

Both sublingual and swallowed tablets are the most convenient and consistent delivery method available. They are also an excellent option for travel, since the majority of patients have concerns about the legality of marijuana in other states and countries. Traveling with tablets and capsules allows you to be much more discreet. Most people with chronic pain are comfortable with taking pills, and these MMJ tablets are as close as we've come to approximating the pharmaceuticals in both form and consistency. The dosage on the label is exactly what you're getting in each tablet.

Disadvantages of tablets and capsules: As with edibles, there is a risk of taking too much. Since each of us will have a somewhat different reaction, I suggest starting gradually with a low dose, waiting at least two hours to evaluate the effect, then deciding if you need more. The sublingual mints are scored tablets, so they're easy to break in half.

JUICING

Vegetables are defined as "any plant cultivated for food, edible herb or root." Cannabis has been referred to as the "most important vegetable on the planet" because it can strengthen the function of your immune system, provide anti-inflammatory benefits, and improve bone metabolism and nerve function, as well as inhibit cancer cell growth.

Some vegetables may be eaten raw, while others must be cooked in order to be edible. When certain fruits and vegetables are heated, they lose a majority of their beneficial enzymes and nutrients. Cannabis is no different. As an edible herb, it is technically a vegetable, containing many of the same nutrients as other leafy greens (such as fiber, iron, and calcium). But its raw leaves are also filled with beneficial cannabinoids, particularly THCa, CBDa, and CBG (described in Chapter 3). As such, juiced cannabis is a nutritionally dense, very potent medicine without the psychoactive effects one would normally experience when heating the plant.

THCa and CBDa must be heated in order to produce THC and CBD. However, according to Dr. William Courtney, a dietary raw cannabis specialist and a strong proponent of the plant's medicinal benefits, "you are actually walking away from 99 percent of the benefits cannabis provides when you cook or smoke cannabis."

Additionally, the body is able to tolerate larger dosages of cannabinoids when cannabis is consumed in the raw form. Your body can only absorb approximately ten milligrams of THC at a time when you smoke cannabis. According to Dr. Courtney, "If you don't heat marijuana, you can go up to five or six hundred milligrams and use the plant strictly as a dietary supplement by upping the antioxidant and neuro-protective levels which come into play at hundreds of milligrams of CBDa and THCa. It is this dramatic increase in dose from 10 mg of psychoactive THC to the 500 mg to 1000 mg of non-psychoactive THCa, CBDa, and CBGa that comprises the primary difference between traditional medical marijuana treatments and using cannabis as a dietary supplement."

The FDA has recently approved a tolerable CBD dose of 600 mg per day as a new investigative drug. This makes the medical potential of drinking the juice containing 600 mg of CBDa far greater than when you heat cannabis. Considering that CBD percentages are typically below 1 percent in most strains available in dispensaries, it is nearly impossible to smoke enough in one day to ingest a 600 mg dosage of CBD.

If you're interested in juicing marijuana, Dr. Courtney recommends that patients juice fifteen leaves and two large (two to four inches long) raw buds per day. Raw buds are flowers harvested when the THC glands are clear (rather than amber). Be aware that this juice is highly acidic and has a bitter taste, and should therefore be diluted either with water or preferably with another type of vegetable or fruit juice (a ratio of one part cannabis juice to ten parts other juice is recommended). Both organic apple and carrot juice are popular choices. There are many good recipes for juicing online.

Split the juice drink into three parts and drink one with each meal, or store it for up to three days in a tightly sealed container in the refrigerator.

Advantages of juicing: An excellent and discreet method for deriving both the health and medicinal benefits of cannabis without the psychoactive and other negative effects of smoking or vaporizing. Juicing is especially effective for inflammatory conditions such as osteoarthritis, rheumatoid arthritis, colitis, Crohn's, and other autoimmune conditions.

Juicing cannabis is also a good preventive medicine, infusing the body with vitamins, minerals, and phytochemicals—natural compounds occurring only in plants that can aid human health by guarding against chronic illness. There are an abundance of phytochemicals in every healthy fruit and vegetable, and they convey antioxidant and even anti-cancer properties.

Disadvantages of juicing: Juicing requires raw, freshly picked, and properly grown cannabis free of any pesticides or other microbiological contaminants. Unless you grow your own plants, this is not easy to find. A few dispensaries do provide fresh cannabis for juicing, but not many. Marijuana that has been dried and prepared for smoking is not suitable for juicing.

TOPICALS

Topicals are cannabis-infused products that are absorbed through the skin for both *localized* and *generalized* relief of pain, soreness, and inflammation.

Localized Topicals

These include *creams*, *lotions*, *balms*, *sprays*, and *oils*. Because they're non-psychoactive, localized topicals are an excellent choice for patients who want pain relief without the psychoactive effect associated with most of the other delivery methods, including the generalized topicals.

Localized topicals are applied directly to the skin covering the area of pain. Their primary active ingredients are CBD, THCa, and CBC (non-psychoactive potent anti-inflammatories), as well as other cannabinoids. They often contain other ingredients, such as arnica (a homeopathic remedy for pain and inflammation) and essential oils to enhance pain relief, such as cayenne, peppermint, wintergreen, and clove. They work by binding to the network of CB2 receptors found throughout the body. These receptors are activated either by the body's naturally occurring endocannabinoids or by cannabis compounds known as phytocannabinoids (e.g., THC, CBD). Even if a topical contains active THC, it's usually a very small amount and won't induce the psychoactive effect.

A localized topical I've found to be one of the most consistently effective for relieving my patients' pain is Apothecanna Extra Strength. It's a double strength moisturizing body cream with anti-inflammatory plant extracts, containing CBD, arnica, peppermint (cooling and anti-inflammatory), and juniper (antiseptic and antirheumatic). Apothecanna Extra Strength provides fast-acting relief from pain and inflammation, in addition to moisturizing and cooling dry and irritated skin. It can be applied directly to sore muscles and painful joints or used as a full body massage.

I always recommend this topical to patients with arthritis, postoperative pain, and chronic pain resulting from serious injuries. I've known several patients who have used Apothecanna to successfully treat their *migraine headaches* by applying it to both temples and forehead, just between the eyebrows. I've not heard that about any other topical.

I've also seen several women who have successfully treated their *menstrual cramps* by applying Apothecanna cream to their lower abdomen/pelvic area, directly over their uterus. It was initially quite surprising to me that this topical has the capacity and potency to penetrate deeply enough to pass through several layers of body tissue, including the skin, fat, and abdominal muscles, to reach and then be absorbed into the uterine muscles where it relieves the cramping.

Another highly effective localized topical is Mary's Medicinals CBC Transdermal Compound. This is the first topical cream on the market that isolates the cannabinoid CBN (well known for its analgesic properties). Immediate benefits include relief from inflammation of the joints and skin irritation, as well as antibacterial properties. These two localized topicals have frequently been reported by my patients to work extremely well for pain relief, but there are a number of others, especially Restore Relief (from Restorative Botanicals), with similar pain-relieving properties, containing cannabinoids along with other analgesic and anti-inflammatory ingredients.

High-CBD hash oils are another effective topical option, especially for *killing cancer cells* when applied on a daily (or twice daily) basis directly to the skin cancer, whether it's a melanoma or a basal or squamous cell carcinoma. (A study that was published in the *Journal of Clinical Investigation* in 2003 found that the cannabinoids in marijuana stop the growth of skin cancer cells.) However, with any of these skin cancers, the topical should be used as a complement to conventional cancer treatment. They've also been helpful in treating *psoriasis*, *eczema*, and other forms of dermatitis. Although I've not worked with any patients who have tried it, I would recommend it for treating actinic keratosis, considered a precancerous lesion, and warts as well.

Cannabis-infused massage oils containing cooling menthol or peppermint are excellent topicals to use both prior to and following a strenuous workout or for sore and aching muscles in general.

Advantages of localized topicals: They provide pain relief where you need it most, without a psychoactive effect. They are effective, convenient, discreet, and can be used any time of day, especially while working. Their effectiveness—without getting high—makes them the preferred daytime medical marijuana product for many of my chronic pain patients, especially those with neck, back, and joint pain.

Disadvantages of localized topicals: They are expensive and their duration of action is relatively short, approximately two hours. This results in frequent reapplication, and if the topicals are used daily, containers are emptied rather quickly.

Generalized Topicals—Transdermals

Generalized topicals differ from localized as a result of the cannabinoids being absorbed directly into the bloodstream (they're applied to the wrist) and therefore affecting the entire body.

The generalized topicals I recommend to patients are Mary's Medicinals Transdermal Gel Pens and Mary's Medicinals Transdermal Patches. There are four types of the unique five-inch, cylindrical transdermal *pens*. Each of them releases a 2 mg dose of CBD, or CBN, with a THC Indica–THC Sativa, turn-click system. The gel is applied to the forearm and is distinguished from other topicals in the fast and complete absorption of the compound into the bloodstream. Patients with generalized pain, such as fibromyalgia, seem to benefit most from the pens.

There are several varieties of the two- by two-inch-square adhesive transdermal *patches*: CBD, 1:1/CBD:THC, THCa, indica, sativa, and CBN. They are the first of their kind on the market and use the unique delivery method of venous absorption. Patients are instructed to apply them to either their wrist or ankle, where the skin is thin and the veins are close to the surface. Patches can be worn for up to twelve hours of continuous effect. If the patient no longer wishes to feel the effect for whatever reason, the patch can be removed and the effect will dissipate within approximately one half hour.

I've had good results with the 1:1/CBD:THC for pain relief, the THCa patch for inflammation, the CBN for sleep and pain, and the CBD for reducing anxiety. Patients who are interested in consuming either an indica or a sativa will usually prefer other delivery methods, especially vaporizing flower.

Advantages of transdermals: Pain relief without inhalation and duration of action (ten to twelve hours), especially with the patches, are the primary advantages. The 1:1/CBD:THC has been an excellent choice for many of my elderly patients with chronic pain, especially those with arthritis. They do not want to inhale, and the psychoactive effect with the patch seems a bit milder, with a slower onset, than with the other delivery methods. The patches are also useful for terminal patients and hospice care. Both pens and patches are convenient and discreet.

Disadvantages of transdermals: Not as effective for severe pain as most of the other delivery methods. They are expensive.

As you can see from both this and the preceding chapter, there are a great many available options for consuming medical marijuana. The challenge is to find the best combination of MMJ product and delivery system to meet your specific needs, and one that works in harmony with your unique body, without causing discomfort. In these two chapters, I have provided you with sufficient information to make well-informed choices to begin the process of selecting the delivery method(s) that works best for you. This might entail a brief (two- to three-week) period of experimentation. I suggest you try several of these methods at least twice while varying the dose of the MMJ to determine the ideal formula for you. With a multitude of options for pain relief and relatively few adverse side effects with short-term daily use, I'm confident you will be successful. Enjoy the process!

Now that you've read Part I, consider yourself a knowledgeable patient and well prepared to begin using cannabis as medicine. Part II will assist you in the process of integrating this knowledge into a holistic treatment program for significantly relieving your pain and treating your specific chronic condition. And if you choose to go further, Part III will reveal how this remarkable herbal medicine can help you to further address the *causes of your dis-ease* and *heal your life*.

PART II
Self-Care 101

MMJ + Holistic Medicine = Long-Lasting Pain Relief

Introduction to Part II

Part II provides additional guidance for using MMJ to treat the most common chronic pain conditions. Patients challenged with a diagnosis other than those presented in Part II can begin applying what they learned in Part I. If possible you can also use the recommendations for a similar condition, or those listed in Chapter 5, "Inflammation," to obtain significant pain relief.

Once you are feeling as if the pain is under reasonably good control and is no longer a major distraction or the central focus of your life, you may be interested in taking the next steps toward long-lasting pain relief. In addition to "Medical Marijuana Recommendations," which discusses the products, strains, and delivery methods most effective for every condition, each chapter in Part II includes "Holistic Medical Treatment and Prevention (HMTP)." By adhering to this treatment program, you should be able to reduce consumption of MMJ from daily (or multiple times per day) to less frequent use.

As you learned in Part I, there can be unpleasant psychological consequences to daily use of marijuana, especially with high-THC (sativa) or even moderate-THC (hybrid) products. The evidence indicates a significant link between daily use of cannabis and *depression, memory loss, cognitive impairment* (including the inability to discriminate time intervals and space distances), and *information processing*. From my own observation and that of many psychotherapists, I would add *anxiety, impulsivity, irritability*, and *anger* to this list of symptoms. Depression is associated with low levels of dopamine (a chemical in the body responsible for feelings of pleasure), and although an immediate effect of THC is an increase in dopamine, *chronic use of marijuana causes the brain to reduce dopamine* production. The decreased dopamine might then trigger a need for more marijuana to relieve the depression, thus creating a dependence that can be both behavioral and physical. Seven to 10 percent of daily users will develop dependence.

Part II, especially the HMTP Program, will help you to avoid dependence by addressing the causes of your chronic pain, thus reducing the need for MMJ. "Getting high" is a pleasurable habit, but if this medicine is not needed for pain relief, then daily use is *excessive* and can become a problem. It may manifest as a subtle change in behavior that you're not even aware of, but which is often obvious to your spouse or partner. As your pain subsides, I would suggest gradually reducing your use of marijuana to two to three times per week; and even less frequently if there is further resolution. One of the rules that I live by, for experiencing a state of optimal health: *Everything in moderation, including moderation.*

In the HMTP section of each chapter you will also find the following subsections: "Risk Factors and Causes"; "Physical Health Recommendations," including diet, vitamins, supplements, and herbs; and "The Issues in Your Tissues: Mental and Emotional Health Recommendations," which highlight beliefs, attitudes, and emotions associated with your specific condition. Rather than merely relieving symptoms temporarily, holistic medicine is largely a self-care practice focused on identifying and addressing each of the underlying causes of your disease. These might be dietary, anatomical/postural, environmental, mental, emotional, or spiritual factors that manifest as pain or dysfunction in your body. By treating each of the contributors to your pain, you will be practicing whole-person, *holistic*, or body-mind-spirit medicine. This practice is essential not only for longer-lasting pain relief, but especially if you're interested in *preventing* recurrences or flare-ups of your pain, possibly *curing* the chronic condition, and leading a vibrantly healthy life. I call it *fully alive medicine.*

The HMTP Program, with MMJ as an integral component, is a healing and spiritual growth process that begins with your commitment to become a much better caretaker of yourself. Think of it as taking on a new full-time job described as: *learning to love and nurture myself at a higher level than I've ever known*. I call it *training to thrive*, and it's been my full-time job since 1980, when at the age of thirty-three I was told I'd have to live with the misery of chronic sinusitis forever. Since then I've cured the sinusitis and have experienced a quality of life I describe as *fully alive*.

The adventure of this lifetime begins by taking your first of many baby steps. I suggest you read the chapter(s) focused on your specific condition(s) as well as Chapters 5 and 15. Chapter 5 addresses *inflammation*, a universal contributor to chronic pain. The MMJ recommendations presented in this chapter can be helpful for treating nearly all of the chronic pain conditions in subsequent chapters.

I would also suggest completing the Candida Questionnaire, before moving on to the chapter with your specific diagnosis. If you find that you are an appropriate candidate for treatment—i.e., you score high on the questionnaire—I recommend you follow through on the Candida Treatment program outlined in Chapter 5, regardless of what your chronic pain condition happens to be. Candida overgrowth is an especially frequent contributor to fibromyalgia, IBS, ulcerative colitis, and Crohn's disease. It can also be a factor contributing to osteoarthritis, as well as depression and insomnia.

The single most important part of Chapter 5 is the *diet*—anti-inflammatory, alkalinizing, candida-controlling, and hypoallergenic. This diet is applicable to nearly all of the conditions included in Part II. Wherever it differs, specific dietary recommendations will be made in the "Diet" section of that chapter.

This is also a healthy, nutritious diet, one that is recommended for anyone interested in optimal health. In addition to what you learn in Chapter 5, you should adhere to the MMJ and holistic medicine recommendations for your particular diagnosis, presented in one of the following chapters.

The most common *emotional pain conditions*—depression, anxiety, and insomnia—are presented in Chapter 15. To some extent, each of us can relate to one or more of these energy-depleting conditions, since most chronic pain patients have some degree of each of these three.

Increased anxiety nearly always accompanies chronic pain, which then contributes to insomnia, and the subsequent sleep-deprivation can increase both depression and anxiety, causing more pain. Fortunately, in most instances it doesn't take long for MMJ to break this debilitating cycle.

After reading Chapter 15, you can begin implementing the recommendations in Part II. Give yourself at least six to eight weeks after beginning the HMTP Program before applying the practices described in Part III. This length of time is needed to be certain that you're maintaining a consistent improvement, and experiencing less pain. The realization that you're actually getting better, after all the months or years of suffering, is a powerful motivator for exploring more deeply the mental, emotional, and spiritual aspects of health presented in Part III.

I advise my patients that a minimum commitment of three months is required to complete the basic HMTP Program (Parts II and III). If you've experienced significant improvement in your physical condition—i.e., your pain has been reduced and you're using less (or no) medication, sleeping better, and have fewer symptoms (other than pain)—you will most likely be interested in continuing with the holistic treatment program.

In order to measure your progress during the first three months, I suggest you maintain a *symptom chart*. I recommend either the one below, which I use in my practice, or you can make your own. When you record the numeric rating of your pain or symptom (0 = no pain or symptom, 10 = incapacitating), you are evaluating your *average* level for that *week*, both *with* and *without* MMJ. The same is true for measuring your ability to function and your mood, sleep (number of hours), and quality of life. For example, if your pain level while using MMJ during that week averages between a 3 or 4, then record it as a 3.5, and if without MMJ it is consistently between a 6 and 8, then record it as a 7. If you are also taking a pain medication or supplements, then they too should be noted on your chart.

For each of the chronic pain conditions, there are *other symptoms* beside pain that will also be affected by MMJ, medication, and/or supplements. Please note these other uncomfortable symptoms on your symptom chart using the same numeric rating system.

Chronic Pain Symptom Chart

Week	1	2	3	4	5	6	7	8	9	10	11	12
Pain with MMJ												
Pain without MMJ												
Function												
Mood												
Hours of Sleep												
Quality of Life												
Other Symptoms												
Medications												
Supplements												

To determine which MMJ products are most effective for you, it is helpful to keep a record of the different products you've used and their effect on your pain. Record your pain level before and after using each product. For example, if your pain is a 9 before vaporizing Harlequin and a 4 after, then record it as 9→ 4. You can use the MMJ log below or create your own.

MMJ Log	
MMJ Product	Date + Effect
Example: Vaporize Harlequin	11/1/17 9 → 4

As you know, cannabis medicine is still in its early infancy. There have been too few studies to *definitively* state that a particular MMJ product works well for treating a specific chronic pain condition. The vast majority of the MMJ recommendations I've made in the following chapters are based on my clinical experience working with more than seven thousand chronic pain patients. I've also received valuable input from the owner and manager of a medical dispensary in Boulder that is establishing the industry standard for dispensaries. They have diligently listened to their customers, recorded their feedback, and continually upgraded their inventory to provide the most therapeutic products for the most common chronic pain conditions, all of which are presented in this book.

By keeping these records, both the symptom chart and the MMJ log, you will have an opportunity to help yourself and millions of others suffering with the same chronic pain condition. If you've had success in relieving your pain with MMJ, and are interested in participating, I'd like you to contact me using the information found in Resources. I will in turn keep you informed via email about the most current information regarding the MMJ products and dietary and supplement recommendations that are the most therapeutic for your specific condition.

The art and science of medicine is continually evolving, and by sending me this information you can help me and many others learn what products are effective in treating the most common chronic pain conditions.

Healing is a dynamic process, one that's unique to each individual. I can help guide you, but it's your level of commitment to the life-changing holistic treatment program outlined in Parts II and III that will determine your degree of success.

I'm well aware that you may have several other full-time jobs—the one from which you earn a living, plus the one you serve as a spouse, parent, or possibly a caretaker of a loved one. We all wear multiple hats. But now I'm asking you to make the *practice of exceptional self-care your highest priority*. Those closest to you will benefit from the depth of this commitment to yourself. Payment for your efforts will not necessarily come with money, although you are quite likely to perform your occupational responsibilities better than you did previously. Your new job will instead reward you with an abundance of vitality, love, happiness, and a heightened sense of being *fully alive*. This is the intended outcome of the practice of holistic medicine, and it is not dependent on whether or not you cure the physical problem.

Part II is essentially a *body-mind quick-fix*. Several of the recommended supplements, especially those from the Metagenics and Xymogen companies, can only be obtained through a health care practitioner. I am making these available in Resources.

As you progress, hope is rekindled. You will become empowered and deepen your commitment to your unique path of self-healing, simply because you are choosing to receive and feel worthy of this degree of nurturing attention from yourself. Part II provides you with an opportunity to practice the art of self-care, with your primary focus on the body and relieving pain.

The art and science of holistic medicine embraces the intimate connection between body, mind, and spirit. As a result of this understanding, for more than forty years the practice of holistic medicine has been remarkably effective for treating, preventing, and often curing *chronic disease*. While conventional medicine has excelled in treating acute and life-threatening illness and injury, it has been largely ineffective for curing chronic ailments, the most common of which is chronic pain. The focus of the holistic practitioner, and my intention for Parts II and III, is to help guide patients and readers to identify the multiple causes of their condition, and work in partnership with them to heal their dis-ease.

The words *heal*, *health*, and *holy* are all derived from the Anglo-Saxon *haelen*. It means "to make whole." *Doctor* is Latin for "*teacher*." As a holistic physician, my job description is literally *teacher of wholeness*.

In America today, there are more than three thousand physicians (MDs and DOs) who have been certified by the American Board of Integrative Holistic Medicine (ABIHM). The foundational beliefs infusing the art, science, and practice of integrative holistic medicine are that *unconditional love is life's most powerful healer*, and its corollary, that *the perceived loss of love is our greatest health risk*. Distilled down to two words: *LOVE HEALS!* And there is no one better suited to dispense that medicine than you.

But I can understand that after reading Part II you might be interested in more personal guidance with the Holistic Medical Treatment and Prevention Program. Fortunately there are enough ABIHM physicians to serve the majority of America's chronic pain sufferers. You can find one near you by going to www.abihm.org and clicking on "Find an ABIHM Certified Physician."

In Part II you will begin to learn the art of nourishing, nurturing, and rejuvenating your body, essentially *loving your dysfunctional body part*. And in Part III I will present you with several healing practices for inspiring your mind, opening your heart, and soothing your soul. Throughout the remainder of the book, medical marijuana will serve you in myriad ways. It is truly a remarkable holistic medicine, one which will facilitate a most enjoyable healing journey!

Patient Story—**Osteoarthritis**

To give you an idea of how life-changing the holistic approach can be, I'll share with you the story of Barbara J., a fifty-two-year-old legal assistant, who came to see me primarily for an MMJ evaluation. A friend with an MMJ card had given her a small amount of an indica strain to smoke for relief of her arthritis pain. Her pain level was consistently between a 4 and a 6 unless she took Celebrex or ibuprofen, in which case it was reduced to between a 2 and a 4. She was concerned about the side effects of these drugs and was shocked at how well the MMJ worked to relieve her pain (reduced it to a 1 to a 2) and helped her to feel better in general (more relaxed, less anxiety).

After smoking it a few times, she decided she wanted to have access to the higher-CBD cannabis products available only at the medical dispensaries. For this she would need a physician recommendation and an MMJ license.

I reviewed her medical history and symptoms, in addition to the diagnosis of osteoarthritis (diagnosed by her primary care physician) and the symptoms of pain and stiffness in her hip, knee, and low back. She also mentioned that she had extreme fatigue, muscle aches, insomnia, moderate depression, and mental fog (inability to concentrate). These latter symptoms made me suspicious of candida overgrowth, and subsequently her score after completing the Candida Questionnaire was 210, in the "Almost certainly yeast-connected" category (see Chapter 5).

After suggesting she try several of the MMJ products in Chapter 6, I also gave Barbara a handout describing the candida-control, antiinflammatory diet and some antifungal supplements and probiotics. In addition I instructed her to begin testing the pH of her urine to monitor her body's level of acidity (higher acidity fuels inflammation).

Barbara returned in six weeks and was quite pleased to report that she felt much better. After a few difficult days during the first week with a die-off reaction (yeast organisms release toxins as they die), she was amazed at how dramatically her overall condition had improved. Her pain level was down to a 2 to a 4 without taking anything (MMJ or the drugs), her energy level had increased from a 3 to a 6, the muscle aching was completely gone, and she was sleeping much better (using MMJ most nights before bed).

At this second visit I presented some of the mental and emotional issues that Louise Hay, author of *You Can Heal Your Life*, believes are connected to arthritis and candidiasis, such as sensitivity to criticism, frustration, and anger. The anger is often directed at oneself in the form of self-criticism. Barbara acknowledged that she was very hard on herself, and was shocked at the accuracy and specificity of this mind-body connection. She left the office with homework to create a short list of affirmations reflecting her goals as the next step on the path toward creating her ideal life.

I recently saw Barbara for the renewal of her MMJ license, one year after her first visit, and she looked noticeably different. There was much more vitality in her face and eyes, she had lost about twenty pounds, and she seemed to be more positive and energetic. She was still taking the maintenance dose of the arthritis supplements and a probiotic daily; she had continued on a somewhat modified (not quite as restrictive) candida-control, anti-inflammatory diet; and she was still using MMJ most nights for sleep, and occasionally during the day (on weekends), simply to get high (not for the purpose of pain relief). Her only occasional symptom was joint pain, which was rarely above a 2 and typically occurred when she was more stressed.

She reported feeling "like a new person." Her energy level was back to normal; she was exercising three to five days a week (without any pain); and she was much happier, with a more positive attitude and a much greater sense of control over her life.

Barbara is an excellent example of a patient who combined MMJ with holistic medicine and obtained a great outcome. She was able to relieve her pain while healing her life.

Chapter 5

Inflammation
Chill Out

Inflammation can be a localized or systemic physical condition in which part(s) of the body become reddened, swollen, hot, and often painful, especially as a reaction to injury or infection. Injury can result from both external (e.g., a fall or overexertion) or internal (e.g., toxins, painful emotions) factors. There are many inflammatory conditions that are systemic—i.e., they affect the whole body. This is especially true of the autoimmune conditions, such as rheumatoid arthritis and systemic lupus erythematosus. There are also instances in which there are overlapping inflammatory conditions occurring at the same time, such as fibromyalgia and osteoarthritis.

MEDICAL MARIJUANA RECOMMENDATIONS FOR INFLAMMATION

- THCa tincture: THCa is the most potent anti-inflammatory of all the cannabinoids, and tincture is the most effective way to administer it. Many patients also use THCa tincture preventively for inflammation.
- High-CBD strains of flower: Harlequin (a 50:50/S:I hybrid), Lucy (a 70:30/I:S indica), and Cannatonic (a 50:50 hybrid).
- High-CBD tinctures: 1:1, 2:1, 3:1, 6:1, or 20:1/CBD:THC.
- High-CBD hash oil: 3:1, 6:1, or 20:1/CBD:THC. The 20:1 hash oil, if available, has been effective in some instances in which THCa tincture was not.

- 3:2/CBDa:THCa transdermal patch
- THCa transdermal patch
- 1:1/CBD:THC transdermal patch
- Indica strains of flower
- Indica and hybrid edibles
- Any strain or MMJ product containing CBG. I found one local MMJ dispensary that had a high-CBG indica strain called Permafrost, a 70:30/I:S.

NOTE: Use caution with sativa strains and high-THC products: Although THC has anti-inflammatory properties and can be useful to some patients, it can also increase anxiety, which has the potential to increase inflammation.

HOLISTIC MEDICAL TREATMENT AND PREVENTION PROGRAM FOR INFLAMMATION AND CANDIDA OVERGROWTH

Physical Health Recommendations

Nearly all chronic pain is accompanied by some degree of inflammation. The foundation for holistically treating inflammatory conditions is an anti-inflammatory diet. You can't expect to manage or overcome chronic pain if you are eating a diet that is fueling chronic inflammation. The majority of Americans are eating 160 pounds of sugar a year, 200 pounds of unhealthy fats, excess refined carbohydrates, and too few vegetables, and are generally eating too much junk.

Inflammation is often fueled by higher levels of acidity, food allergies, candida overgrowth, and increased anxiety. *Diet* can profoundly impact each of these factors. This is the reason for recommending the following *anti-inflammatory, alkalinizing, candida-control,* and *hypoallergenic* diet. I call it the **Fully Alive Diet**, since it can play such a pivotal role in experiencing optimal health.

As I have previously mentioned, MMJ is effective for pain relief and pain management. But the anti-inflammatory diet is critical for long-term reduction of the underlying causes of inflammation, which can dramatically lessen inflammatory-based symptoms. Since this basic diet can be applied to treating most of the conditions in Part II, I am presenting it here rather than including it in each of the subsequent chapters. Regardless of what pain condition you are experiencing, I urge you to seriously consider making a commitment to following these dietary instructions to get the best outcome you can.

After reviewing the diet, you may be thinking, "There is nothing for me to eat." You may not find your favorite foods on this diet, but I can assure you there are plenty of nutritious and appetizing options from which to choose. There are also several good cookbooks available at most health food stores. I recommend *The Candida Cure Cookbook: Delicious Recipes to Reset Your Health and Restore Your Vitality*, by Ann Boroch, and *Erica White's Beat Candida Cookbook*, by Erica White.

If you can closely adhere to the dietary recommendations for at least the first month, you should notice a definite improvement in your pain level, *even without medical marijuana*. If this is the case, then you can loosen the dietary restrictions just a bit, and see how your body responds.

Anti-Inflammatory, Alkalinizing, Candida-Control, and Hypoallergenic Diet

Foods to Include—First Twenty-One Days

> *Vegetables*: Eat freely; 50 to 60 percent of total diet; raw or lightly steamed; organic and clean (wash well); high-water-content and low-starch vegetables (3 percent and 6 percent on glycemic index are best— refer to "Glycemic Index" on page 104 and "Carbohydrate Classification of Fruits and Vegetables" on page 105).

> - *Green leafy*: all lettuce, spinach, parsley, cabbage, kale, collard greens, watercress, beet greens, mustard greens, bok choy, sprouts
> - *Low starch*: celery, zucchini, summer squash, crookneck squash, green beans, broccoli, cauliflower, brussels sprouts, radishes, bell pepper (green, red, yellow), asparagus, cucumber, tomato, onion, leek, garlic, kohlrabi
> - *Moderately low starch*: carrots, beets, rutabaga, turnip, parsnip, eggplant, artichoke, avocado, water chestnuts, peas (green, snow peas), okra

Protein: Emphasis at breakfast and lunch with no less than sixty grams per day; meats should be antibiotic- and hormone-free; fish should be fresh deepwater ocean fish; seeds and nuts should be raw and organic. Acceptable proteins include: fresh ocean fish (salmon, sole, cod, halibut), canned fish (salmon, sardines, and tuna—no more than two times per week), turkey, ground turkey, chicken, lamb, wild game, Cornish hens, eggs (especially organic, free-range, high-omega-3-fat yolks—limit two to four per week), seeds and nuts (almonds, cashews, pecans, filberts, pine nuts, Brazil nuts, walnuts, pistachios, pumpkin seeds, sunflower seeds, sesame seeds—raw and unsalted).

Complex carbohydrates: whole grains (non-gluten is preferable); eat only enough to maintain your energy (try to limit yourself to one serving or half a cup a day or less); restriction varies according to food allergy, which can be determined with an elimination diet (see page 108).

Non-gluten grains: brown rice, millet, quinoa, buckwheat, and amaranth; eat sprouted or cooked; organic and clean; available in bulk at health food stores; rotate grains every four days; tasty as breakfast cereals, in salads and soups, in casseroles and stir-frys; store away from light and heat in airtight containers; other whole grains (*with gluten*) that should be eaten in *only limited amounts* include barley, spelt, wild rice, corn, oats, cornmeal, bulgur, and couscous.

NOTE: Flour of any kind, whole grain or not, may be high glycemic (rapidly increasing your blood sugar load), which creates a surge of insulin that might increase inflammation. During the first twenty-one days, try avoiding flour products in general and then minimize after that. See page 104.

Oils: flaxseed, avocado, raw coconut, extra virgin olive oil—1 to 2 tablespoons daily; use on grains or vegetables or as a salad dressing; as much as possible do not heat or cook with these oils, although cooking with olive or coconut oil is OK in moderation; keep flax oil refrigerated and away from light; other acceptable oils (cold-pressed) are walnut and macadamia nut; use within six weeks of opening.

After 21 Days

Fruits: Introduce fruits into your diet slowly, limiting yourself to one serving per day until you are sure they do not make your symptoms worse. Start with melons, berries (blueberries, raspberries, huckleberries, blackberries), lemons and grapefruit, and other fruits on the 3 percent "Glycemic Index" list (only after first twenty-one days of the diet); then choose from among most other fresh fruits, all of which are generally sweeter than the first group. These include apple, pear, peach, orange, nectarine, apricot, cherry, and pineapple. Fruit juices should be very diluted, at least 1:1 with water. Freshly squeezed is best. Avoid full-strength fruit juices, canned fruit juices, and all dried fruits.

Complex carbohydrates: Starchy vegetables and legumes.

Starchy vegetables: new and red potatoes, sweet potatoes, yams, winter squash (acorn, butternut), pumpkin, Yukon Gold potatoes

Legumes: lentils, split peas, black-eyed peas, beans (kidney, garbanzo, black, navy, pinto, lima, adzuki)

Fermented yeast- and mold-containing foods: These are allowable only if you're not allergic. However, I would introduce them very gradually (eat a particular food no more than once every three to four days) and do not begin until you have been on the diet for at least three weeks. These foods include: fermented dairy products such as yogurt, kefir, buttermilk, low-fat cottage cheese, and sour cream; fermented foods such as sauerkraut, kimchi, fermented vegetables, tofu, tempeh, miso, and soy sauce.

NOTE: If you have chronic sinus or respiratory problems, avoid *all* dairy products.

Seed/nut butters: raw almond butter, raw sesame tahini, raw pumpkin seed butter, raw walnut butter, raw filbert butter, raw sunflower seed butter

GLYCEMIC INDEX

Carbohydrates act like a powerful drug elevating insulin in the body. This in turn can increase fat deposits, LDL cholesterol (the unhealthy kind), and inflammation, while decreasing immunity. The amount of insulin the body produces is based on the amount of carbohydrate that actually enters the bloodstream as the simple sugar glucose. This is why you can consume a large amount of the 3 percent or 6 percent vegetables and fruits (refer to "Carbohydrate Classifications of Fruits and Vegetables") in comparison to the amount of grains, starches, breads, or pastas at any given meal (*example*: 1½ cups of broccoli, or any other 3 percent vegetable = ¼ cup pasta).

It is best to focus on the low-density carbohydrates (3 percent and 6 percent). Not only can you eat more, but there are many other benefits, including high water content, high fiber content, vitamins, minerals, and enzymes. People are genetically designed to eat primarily fruits and vegetables as their major source of carbohydrates.

All carbohydrates, simple or complex, have to be broken down into simple sugars before being absorbed by the body and entering the bloodstream. The only simple sugar that can actually enter the bloodstream is glucose. The faster glucose enters the bloodstream, the more insulin you make. This is important for you to know when you are making your choice of carbohydrates. *The higher the glycemic index of a carbohydrate, the faster it enters the bloodstream as sugar.*

Low Glycemic Index Foods (3 percent and 6 percent fruits and vegetables)

- Fructose has to be converted into glucose via the liver, so fruits have a lower glycemic index than grains and starches. Three to eight cups of 3 to 6 percent vegetables per day are recommended, as well as two to three servings of 3 to 6 percent fruits (1 cup = 1 serving).

High Glycemic Index Foods (bagel, pasta, cooked starches)

- Cornflakes are pure glucose linked by chemical bonds. These bonds are easily broken in the stomach and glucose rushes into the bloodstream.

Table sugar is one half glucose and one half fructose, so it actually enters the bloodstream slower than a bagel.

- There are other factors involved that have an effect on how fast the carbohydrates are broken down into simple sugar. Fat and soluble fibers slow the entry of glucose, and this is an important distinction. There are two types of fiber, soluble (pectin, apples) and insoluble (cellulose and bran cereal). And because fat slows down the entry of glucose into the bloodstream, the sugar in ice cream actually is absorbed more slowly than that of a bagel. High-fiber, low-glycemic foods are the slowest to release sugars.
- The more the carbohydrates are cooked, the higher the glycemic index will be. This is because the cell structure is broken down by cooking and processing. The glycemic index is dramatically increased in instant foods like rice and potatoes.

Highest Glycemic Index Foods (puffed cereal and puffed rice cakes)

- The body needs a constant intake of carbohydrates for optimal brain function. Too much carbohydrate and the body increases insulin secretion to drive down blood sugar. Too little and the brain will not function efficiently. High-glycemic food should always be avoided with candida overgrowth.
- Remember, protein stimulates glucagon, which reduces insulin secretion, while fat and fiber slow down the rate of entry of any carbohydrate.

Carbohydrate Classifications of Fruits and Vegetables (according to carbohydrate content)			
Vegetables			
3%	6%	15%	20%
asparagus	beans, string	artichoke	beans, dried
bean sprouts	beets	carrot	beans, lima
beet greens	brussels sprouts	oyster plant	corn
broccoli	chives	parsnip	potato, sweet
cabbage	collard greens	peas, green	potato, white
cauliflower	dandelion greens	squash	yam

Carbohydrate Classifications of Fruits and Vegetables (according to carbohydrate content)

Vegetables			
3%	6%	15%	20+%
celery	eggplant		
chard, swiss	kale		
cucumber	kohlrabi		
endive	leek		
lettuce	okra		
mustard greens	onion		
radish	parsley		
spinach	peppers, red		
watercress	pimento		
	pimento		
	pumpkin		
	rutabagas		
	turnip		

Fruits			
3%	6%	15%	20+%
cantaloupe	apricots (fresh only)	apples	bananas
rhubarb	blackberries	blueberries	figs
strawberries	cranberries	cherries	prunes
watermelon	grapefruit	grapes	any dried fruit
	guava	kumquats	
	melons	loganberries	
	lemons	mangoes	
	limes	pears	
	oranges	pineapple (fresh)	
	papayas	pomegranates	
	peaches		
	plums		
	raspberries		
	tangerines		

Foods to Avoid

- *Refined sugar and sugar-containing foods*: cakes, cookies, candy, dough-nuts, pastries, ice cream, pudding, soft drinks, pies, etc.; anything containing sucrose (table sugar), fructose, maltose, lactose, glucose, dextrose, corn sweetener, corn syrup, sorbitol, and mannitol; honey; molasses; maple syrup; date sugar; barley malt; rice syrup; NutraSweet and saccharine; table salt (often contains sugar; use sea salt). (To diminish sugar cravings, use chromium bis-glycinate, 200 mcg two times a day; biotin, 500 to 1,000 mcg two times a day; and a methylated B-complex such as B-Activ from Xymogen. Dosage is one capsule two times a day with food—only if you're not already taking a comprehensive multivitamin. Four days without any sugar will also usually eliminate this craving.)
- *Milk and dairy products*: all cheeses (unsweetened soy milk is okay and so is organic butter from grass-fed cows, but not in excess)
- *Bread and other yeast-raised baked items*: including cakes, cookies, and crackers; whole grain cereals; pastas; tortillas; waffles; muffins
- *Beef and pork*
- *Mushrooms*: all types
- *Gluten grains*: wheat, rye, barley, spelt, and oats (there are certified gluten-free oatmeal—e.g., Bob's Red Mill—and granolas; avoid for first three weeks)
- *Fresh fruit* (avoid for first three weeks) and *canned fruit and canned vegetables*
- *Alcoholic beverages*: especially fermented—e.g., beer and wine (alcohol is inflammatory; fermented alcohol is the worst for aggravating candida)
- *Caffeine*: one to two cups of organic coffee a day are okay (Coffee is acidic; green tea is an acceptable substitute)
- *White or refined flour products*: packaged/processed and refined foods
- *Fried foods, fast foods, sausage, and hot dogs*
- *Vinegar, mustard, ketchup, sauerkraut, olives, and pickles* (raw apple cider vinegar is allowed)
- *Margarine, preservatives* (check frozen vegetables)
- *Refined* and hydrogenated oils
- *Leftovers* (freeze them for a later date)
- *Rice milk*: high carbohydrate content

This diet is meant to be a guide. The responses to it will vary greatly depending on the severity of the inflammation, yeast overgrowth, food allergies, and the type of medication (if any) or anti-inflammatory or antifungal supplements you may be taking to reduce inflammation and candida. The majority of people who closely adhere to the diet will experience a significant improvement within one month.

If you've followed this diet for three to four weeks in addition to taking the dietary supplements I've recommended and see no improvement, then I'd recommend going back to the basic vegetable (low-starch) and protein diet and being suspicious of a food allergy. The food you're allergic to is often something you eat every day and have developed a craving for.

Food Elimination for Food Allergy Detection

If you reintroduce new foods very gradually, one new food every three to four days, then you should be able to detect the offending food from the symptoms that arise after eating it. Please pay close attention to your pain (or other symptoms, such as gas, bloating, diarrhea, headache, urinary frequency, nasal congestion) in the first few hours following the introduction of a new food. This trial-and-error method is a simple way to determine food allergies and sensitivities.

Acid/Alkaline Dietary Balance for Pain Reduction

When you are first starting to change your diet and reduce inflammation, it is vital to eat in a way that makes your body more alkaline, rather than acidic. The standard American diet (SAD) tends to be highly acidic. The combination of sugar, coffee, fried fat, excess meat, grain-based carbohydrates, additives, and carbonated sodas contributes too many metabolic acids and increases the acidity of your tissues; i.e., a pH below 7.0. This is especially true if you are over forty years of age. High acidity wreaks havoc on your tissues, by increasing inflammation, slowing down your ability to detoxify, and slowing your metabolism. The result is increased pain!

This occurs as a result of high acidity interfering with optimal enzyme activity throughout the body. You have hundreds of enzymes performing countless functions in your cells every moment of every day. These enzymes depend on a multitude of vitamins and nutrients to function normally, but they are not able to utilize these nutrients in an acidic environment. Your body cannot "water down the fire" of inflammation because these enzymes aren't working properly.

The Fully Alive Diet I've outlined above is naturally more alkalinizing because it emphasizes a high vegetable intake that neutralizes acids with minerals such as potassium, magnesium, calcium, and sodium. You can easily measure if you are more acidic or alkaline by using pH paper test strips that you can find in most pharmacies or health food stores. You can measure either urine or saliva. I think urine is a bit more accurate. The goal is to raise your body's pH to a slightly alkaline level—7.0 to 7.4 is the optimal range. If you start eating a more alkaline diet and your pH continues to measure 6.2 or below, you should seek a personalized program with a holistic medicine professional.

I suggest you measure your pH every day for the first thirty to ninety days of your dietary changes and record the numbers. The numbers can quickly go to the acidic side of the scale if you get too far off your dietary program. You can learn from this, adjust your dietary choices back to the more alkaline side, and watch the pH number get back to 7 or more. Most likely you will feel much better as you stay in this range.

The "Acid/Alkaline Food Chart" on the following pages was created by Russell Jaffe, MD. It is also available online at http://www.drrusselljaffe .com/alkaline-food-chart/.

Cannabis and Acidity

Although it is well known that several of the cannabinoids are anti-inflammatory (e.g., CBD, THCa, CBG), THC is in fact *weakly acidic*. I would only be concerned about it affecting your body's pH if you are using high-THC products multiple times per day, which I'm not recommending for treating chronic pain.

Vitamins and Supplements for Inflammation

Since the majority of chronic pain conditions involve inflammation, I will mention the specific anti-inflammatory vitamins and supplements targeted to each of the conditions in the following chapters.

However, the following four dietary supplements are recommended for anyone suffering with significant inflammation. They should be taken

Food and Chemical Effects on Acid/Alkaline Body Chemical Balance

<<<<
MORE ACID
(Consume Less)

Food Category				
Citrus Fruit Fruit		Cranberry Pomegranate	Plum Prune Tomato	Coconut Fig Guava Persimmon Juice Cherimoya Date Dry Fruit

Bean
Vegetable
Legume
Pulse
Root
	Soybean
	Carob
		Pea Green
		     Snow
		Peanut
		Legumes (other)
		Carrot
		Chick Pea/Garbanzo
			Bean Pinto
			    White
			    Navy/Red
			    Aduki
			    Lima or Mung
			Chard
			Split Pea
				Bean Fava
				    Kidney
				    Black-eyed
				    String/Wax
				Spinach
				Zucchini
				Chutney
				Rhubarb

Grain
Cereal
Grass
	Barley
	Processed Flour
		Corn
		Rye
		Oat Bran
			Wheat Semolina
			    Spelt, teff
			    Kamut
			White Rice
			Buckwheat
				Triticale
				Brown Rice
				Millet
				Kasha

Fowl	Pheasant	Chicken	Goose/Turkey	Wild Duck
Meat Game Fish/Shell Fish	Beef Shell Fish (Processed) Lobster	Pork/Veal Mussel/Squid	Lamb/Mutton Game Meat Shell Fish (Whole)	Gelatin/Organs Venison Fish
Egg				Egg, Chicken
Processed Dairy Cow/Human Soy Goat/Sheep	*Processed Cheese* Ice Cream	Casein Cottage Cheese Milk, Soy	Milk; Goat, Cow, Sheep	Cream/Butter Yogurt Cheese; Goat, Sheep

Oil
Seed/Sprout
Nut
	Cottonseed Oil/Meal
	Fried Food
	Hazelnut
	Walnut
	Brazil Nut
		Oil Chestnut
		    Palm Kernel
		Lard
		Pistachio Seed
		Pecan
			Oil Almond
			    Sesame
			    Safflower
			Tapioca
			Seitan or Tofu
				Oil Canola
				    Pumpkin Seed
				    Grape Seed
				    Sunflower
				Pine Nut

Beverage Preservative Sweetener Vinegar	*Beer* *"Soda"* *Table Salt* Yeast/Hops/Malt *Sugar*/Cocoa White/Acetic Vinegar	Coffee Aspartame Saccharin Red Wine Vinegar	Alcohol Black Tea Benzoate Balsamic Vinegar	Kona Coffee MSG Honey/Maple Syrup Rice Vinegar
Spice/Herb	Pudding/Jam/Jelly	Nutmeg	Vanilla Stevia	Curry
Therapeutic	*Antibiotics*	*Psychotropics*	*Antihistamines*	

Food and Chemical Effects on Acid/Alkaline Body Chemical Balance

>>>> MORE ALKALINE
(Consume More)

⊕	⊕⊕	⊕⊕⊕	⊕⊕⊕⊕	Food Category
Orange Banana Blueberry Raisin, Grapes Currant Strawberry	Lemon Pear Avocado Apple Blackberry Cherry Peach	Grapefruit Canteloupe Honeydew Olive Mango Citrus Loganberry	Lime Nectarine Raspberry Watermelon Tangerine Pineapple	Citrus Fruit Fruit
Brussel Sprout Beet Chive/Scallion Celery/Cilantro Squash Artichoke Lettuce Jicama Turnip Greens	Potato/Bell Pepper Mushroom/Fungi Cauliflower Cabbage Eggplant Pumpkin Collard Greens	Kohlrabi Parsnip/Taro Garlic Asparagus Kale/Parsley Endive/Arugula Jerusalem Artichoke Ginger Root Broccoli	Lentil Brocoflower Seaweed Nori‖Kombu‖ Wakame‖Hijiki‖ Onion/Miso Daikon/Taro Root Sea Vegetables Burdock/Lotus Root Sweet Potato/Yam	Bean Vegetable Legume Pulse Root
Quinoa Wild Rice Oat				Grain Cereal Grass
				Fowl
				Meat Game Fish/Shell Fish
Egg, Duck	Egg, Quail			Egg
Ghee Human Breast Milk				Processed Dairy Cow/Human Soy Goat/Sheep
Oil Avocado Coconut Olive/Macadamia Linseed/Flax Seeds (most)	Oil Cod Liver Primrose Sesame Seed Almond Sprout	Poppy Seed Pepper Chestnut Cashew	Pumpkin Seed	Oil Seed/Sprout Nut
Ginger Tea *Sulfite* Sucanat Umeboshi Vinegar	Green or Mu Tea Rice Syrup Apple Cider Vinegar	Kambucha Molasses Soy Sauce	Mineral Water Sea Salt	Beverage Preservative Sweetener Vinegar
White Willow Bark Slippery Elm Artemesia Annua	Herbs Aloe Vera Nettle	Spices/Cinnamon Valerian Licorice Agave	Baking Soda	Spice/Herb
Algae, Blue Green	Sake		Umeboshi Plum	Therapeutic

Italicized items are NOT recommended

on a daily basis and can be purchased through the professional websites
listed in the Resources section.

- *Multivitamin/mineral/antioxidant/phytonutrient blend*: Most multi-vitamins on the commercial market are not recommended due to their lack of quality control and the fact that they do not incorporate the most recent scientific research. I recommend PhytoMulti from Metagenics. The recommended dosage is one tablet two times a day with food.
- *Fish oil—EPA/DHA*: There are several thousand research papers on fish oil reducing inflammation. Unless you are vegetarian, I recommend Metagenics' OmegaGenics EPA-DHA 720 to all of my patients. It is an extremely high-quality fish oil, and the recommended dosage is two to four capsules a day with food, but only take four capsules daily for two months, then reduce to two capsules a day.
- *Vitamin D3*: With chronic pain, you should have a vitamin D blood level of approximately 70 to 80 ng/ml. Ask your doctor to measure it. I recommend taking at least 5,000 IU daily with food. Optimizing your vitamin D levels is essential in reducing pain. There are several good options for 5,000-unit Vitamin D3 capsules at most health food stores.
- *Probiotic*: There is a great deal of research demonstrating that having a wide diversity of the appropriate species of beneficial bacteria in your intestine can reduce toxins that are absorbed in the gut and trigger inflammation. If you score high on the Candida Questionnaire below, then take the recommended probiotics that are listed in the treatment plan. If not, an excellent daily probiotic with seven highly researched strains is Metagenics' Ultraflora Spectrum. The recommended dosage is one capsule before bed on an empty stomach.

The Issues in Your Tissues: Mental and Emotional Health Recommendations

Louise Hay, in *You Can Heal Your Life*, lists as the probable emotional cause of inflammation: "Fear. Seeing red. Inflamed thinking." The affirmation she recommends for reducing inflammation: *My thinking is peaceful, calm, and centered.*

Many inflammatory conditions end with the suffix "itis." For example, arthritis, colitis, tendinitis. Ms. Hay believes the probable emotional cause of *itis* diagnoses is: "Anger and frustration about conditions you are looking at in your life." Her suggested affirmation: *I am willing to change all patterns of criticism. I love and approve of myself.*

Candida Overgrowth

Yeast is an integral part of life. It is a hardy fungus found in food, air, and on the exposed surfaces of most objects. There are more than 250 species of yeast organisms, and more than 150 of them can be found as harmless parasites in the human body. The most prevalent type of yeast found in and on our bodies is *Candida albicans*. It is an innocuous single-cell fungus and a normal inhabitant of our intestines primarily, and the mouth, respiratory tract, and vagina as well.

Candida is kept under control by the good bacteria that also make their home in the human gastrointestinal, respiratory, and genital tracts. A large percentage of the millions of these friendly bacteria are lactobacillus and bifidus. Similar to the bacteria in yogurt or in raw fermented foods, the lactobacilli make enzymes and vitamins, help fight undesirable bacteria, and lower cholesterol levels. While assisting us in keeping our bowel function and digestion normal, these friendly bacteria, also referred to as acidophilus bacteria, regard candida as their food. Since they are the chief "predator" of candida, they are critical to maintaining a "balance of nature" in our intestines. As long as this homeostatic relationship is maintained, candida poses no problem. However, when an *imbalance* is created and there is an overgrowth or an excessive amount of candida, these organisms then begin secreting *toxins*. This toxicity is a primary cause of the severe inflammation in tissues throughout the body, such as the gastrointestinal tract, respiratory tract, joints, brain, etc.

To an increasing extent, massive overgrowth of candida is resulting in a condition known by a variety of names—candida overgrowth, candidiasis, candida-related complex, candida toxicity syndrome, or as it relates to the sinuses, fungal sinusitis. *The most frequent cause of this imbalance is the recurrent or extended use of antibiotics*, which kill the beneficial bacteria along with those causing the infection for which the antibiotic is being taken. The problem with yeast overgrowth has reached epidemic proportions and is a significant contributing factor to many chronic pain conditions.

Diagnosing Candida Overgrowth

Even in 2017, there is still no consistently reliable laboratory test on which you can always depend to make a definitive diagnosis of candida overgrowth. This is the reason the vast majority of physicians do not believe this condition exists. The diagnostic method I've been using quite effectively for more than twenty years is a combination of obtaining a thorough history, reviewing symptoms, and using Dr. William Crook's Candida Questionnaire and Score Sheet (see below). If you are experiencing several of the possible symptoms, have a story compatible with causing candidiasis, and have a high score on Dr. Crook's questionnaire, there is no laboratory test I'm aware of that is as dependable as this combination for establishing the diagnosis.

Further confirmation can also be obtained via the outcome of antifungal treatment. A significant improvement within three to four weeks of beginning an aggressive treatment program provides excellent confirmation of the diagnosis.

The following is a modification of Dr. William Crook's Questionnaire and Score Sheet that can be used to reliably rule in or rule out the diagnosis of an overgrowth of candida.

CANDIDA QUESTIONNAIRE AND SCORE SHEET

This questionnaire is designed for adults, and the scoring system isn't appropriate for children. It lists factors in your medical history that promote the growth of *Candida albicans* (section A), and symptoms commonly found in individuals with yeast-connected illness (sections B and C).

For each "Yes" answer in Section A circle the point score corresponding to that question, and add your point total and record it at the end of the section. Then move on to Sections B and C and score as directed.

Filling out and scoring the questionnaire should help you and your doctor evaluate the possible role candida plays in contributing to your health problems. Yet it will not provide an automatic yes or no answer.

Section A: Medical History

1. Have you taken tetracyclines (Sumycin, Panmycin, Vibramycin, Minocin, etc.) or other antibiotics for acne for one month or longer?   25

2. Have you, at any time in your life, taken other broad-spectrum antibiotics* for respiratory, urinary, or other infections for two months or longer or in shorter courses four or more times in a one-year period?   20

3. Have you taken a broad-spectrum antibiotic*—even in a single course? 6

4. Have you, at any time in your life, been bothered by persistent prostatitis, vaginitis, or other problems affecting your reproductive organs?   25

5. Have you been pregnant two or more times?   5
   one time?   3

6. Have you taken birth control pills
   for more than two years?   15
   for six months to two years?   8

7. Have you taken prednisone, Decadron, or other cortisone-type drugs, by injection or inhalation
   for more than two weeks?   15
   for two weeks or less?   6

8. Does exposure to perfumes, insecticides, fabric shop odors, and other chemicals provoke
   moderate to severe symptoms?   20
   mild symptoms?   5

---

* Including ampicillin, amoxicillin, Augmentin, Keflex, Ceclor, Bactrim, Septra, Levaquin, Zithromax, and many others. Such antibiotics kill off "good germs" while they are killing off those which cause infection.

9. Are your symptoms worse on damp, muggy days or in moldy places? 20

10. Have you had athlete's foot, ringworm, jock itch, or other chronic fun-
    gus infections of the skin or nails? Have such infections been
    severe or persistent?   20
    mild to moderate?   10

11. Do you crave sugar?   10

12. Do you crave breads?   10

13. Do you crave alcoholic beverages?   10

14. Does tobacco smoke really bother you?   10

TOTAL SCORE, SECTION A: _____

Section B: Symptoms

For each of your symptoms below, enter the point score based on the following:

> Not at all: 0 points
> Occasional or mild: 3 points
> Frequent and/or moderately severe: 6 points
> Severe and/or disabling: 9 points

Add up your total score and record it in the box at the end of this section.

1. Fatigue or lethargy   _____

2. Feeling of being "drained"   _____

3. Poor memory or concentration   _____

4. Feeling "spacey" or "unreal"   _____

5. Depression   _____

6. Numbness, burning, or tingling _____

7. Muscle aches _____

8. Muscle weakness or paralysis _____

9. Pain and/or swelling in joints _____

10. Abdominal pain _____

11. Constipation _____

12. Diarrhea _____

13. Bloating _____

14. Troublesome vaginal discharge _____

15. Persistent vaginal burning or itching _____

16. Prostatitis _____

17. Impotence _____

18. Loss of sexual desire _____

19. Endometriosis or infertility _____

20. Cramps and/or other menstrual irregularities _____

21. Premenstrual tension _____

22. Spots in front of the eyes _____

23. Erratic vision _____

TOTAL SCORE, SECTION B: _____

Section C: Other Symptoms

For each of your symptoms below, enter the point score based on the following:

> Not at all: 0 points
> Occasional or mild: 1 points
> Frequent and/or moderately severe: 2 points
> Severe and/or disabling: 3 points

Add up you total score and record it in the box at the end of this section.

1. Drowsiness   _____

2. Irritability or jitteriness   _____

3. Incoordination   _____

4. Inability to concentrate   _____

5. Frequent mood swings   _____

6. Headache   _____

7. Dizziness/loss of balance   _____

8. Pressure above ears, feeling of head swelling and tingling   _____

9. Itching   _____

10. Other rashes   _____

11. Heartburn   _____

12. Indigestion   _____

13. Belching and intestinal gas _____

14. Mucus in stools _____

15. Hemorrhoids _____

16. Dry mouth _____

17. Rash or blisters in mouth _____

18. Bad breath _____

19. Joint swelling or arthritis _____

20. Nasal congestion or discharge _____

21. Postnasal drip _____

22. Nasal itching _____

23. Sore or dry throat _____

24. Cough _____

25. Pain or tightness in chest _____

26. Wheezing or shortness of breath _____

27. Urinary urgency or frequency _____

28. Burning on urination _____

29. Failing vision _____

30. Burning or tearing of eyes _____

31. Recurrent infections or fluid in ears _____

32. Ear pain or deafness _____

　　TOTAL SCORE, SECTION A: _____
　　TOTAL SCORE, SECTION B: _____
　　TOTAL SCORE, SECTION C: _____
　　GRAND TOTAL SCORE: _____

The Grand Total Score will help you and your doctor decide if your health problems are yeast-connected. Scores in women will run higher as seven items in the questionnaire apply exclusively to women, while only two apply exclusively to men.

If Your Score Is . . .
Greater than:

> 180 (women) or 140 (men)—almost certainly yeast-connected
> 120 (women) or 80 (men)—probably yeast-connected
> 60 (women) or 40 (men)—possibly yeast-connected

Less than:

> 60 (women) or 40 (men)—probably not yeast-connected

Although the diagnostic laboratory tests for candida overgrowth are improving, they have not yet met the current high scientific standards expected for medical diagnosis. This is the primary reason that the majority of physicians fail to recognize the existence of this insidious and debilitating condition.

Candida Treatment Program

- *Candida-control diet* (same as Fully Alive Diet): This diet is the foundation of the holistic treatment program; without good compliance on the diet, the supplements will not be effective.

- *Antifungal supplements*:* The following antifungals should be taken throughout the treatment program (three to six months) in a gradually decreasing dosage.

    1. *AlliMed* (450 mg capsule) or *AlliMax* (180 mg/capsule) are different strengths of the same product—100 percent pure allicin (the active ingredient in garlic). Studies have shown AlliMed to be a highly effective antifungal, antibacterial (kills MRSA, a flesh-eating staph), and antiviral (kills cold viruses), with no adverse side effects (other than its expense). I have been using it in my practice to treat candida overgrowth and fungal sinusitis, to prevent sinus infections and colds, and as a natural "antibiotic" for nearly fifteen years. The recommended dosage (AlliMed): two capsules three times a day for twenty days, then one capsule three times a day for twenty days, then one capsule two times a day for six weeks, then one daily for three months. Can be taken with or without food.

    2. *Candisol* (physician strength) or *Candex* contains an enzyme that destroys the cell wall of the candida organisms and reduces die-off symptoms. It is well tolerated and has become a consistent component of my candida treatment program. The recommended dosage (Candisol or Candex): two capsules morning and night on an empty stomach for three months, then one capsule twice a day for another two to three months. Candex can be found in many health food stores.

    3. *Candicide* is a unique product containing a combination of several antifungal supplements including: sodium caprylate, oregano leaf, pau d'arco, berberine sulfate, and grapefruit seed extract, along with other anti-inflammatory ingredients. Recommended dosage: two capsules three times a day on an empty stomach for two months, then one capsule three times a day for two months, then one capsule two times a day for two months.

    4. *Grapefruit seed extract* in either liquid or capsule (or both) forms is another good antifungal supplement available in nearly all health food stores.

---

* Unless it's mentioned that the product is available in health food stores, all of the products presented in this and the following chapters are available online (see Resources).

- *Probiotics*: These beneficial bacteria are needed to replace the bacteria that have been depleted from your body from a variety of causes, e.g., antibiotics, anti-inflammatories, inflammation. I recommend:

  1. A probiotic containing at least 20 billion organisms, especially lactobacillus acidophilus and bifidus
  2. *Latero-Flora* is a unique strain of bacteria called *Bacillus laterosporus B.O.D.* It has been tested extensively and found to be extremely effective for gastrointestinal dysfunction, food sensitivities, and candidiasis. It also works well as an alkalinizer, and yeast thrives in a more acidic environment.

The Issues in Your Tissues

Louise Hay describes the probable emotional cause of candida overgrowth as: "Feeling very scattered. Lots of frustration and anger. Demanding and untrusting in relationships. Great takers." Her recommended affirmation: *I give myself permission to be all that I can be and I deserve the very best in life. I love and appreciate myself and others.*

I will explain in Chapter 17 how to practice using affirmations along with visualizations to help relieve your pain and heal your life.

The MMJ recommendations in addition to the information about inflammation and candida overgrowth in this chapter can be applied and used as a complement to the treatment recommendations in the following chapters.

Chapter 6

Osteoarthritis and Rheumatoid Arthritis
Love Your Joints

OSTEOARTHRITIS

Osteoarthritis (OA) is the most common form of arthritis, afflicting about 27 million Americans of all ages. It rarely begins before the age of forty, but an estimated 40 to 80 percent of people over the age of sixty-five have some degree of arthritis. The majority of arthritis sufferers do not seek medical treatment. For some people with arthritis, the symptoms remain mild, while in others (about 16 million) symptoms grow progressively worse until they become disabling. Approximately 15 percent of my patients are suffering with osteoarthritis. The most common joints affected by OA are the weight-bearing joints: the knees, hips, and spine. However, there are many people who begin with pain in their thumb and fingers.

Osteoarthritis is an inflammation of the joints that causes a breakdown in the cartilage covering the bone inside the joint. Arthritis usually involves a synovial joint—one that is encased in a tough fibrous capsule lined with a membrane that secretes a thick, clear synovial fluid. This type of joint connects one bone to another and, with the fluid lubricating the cartilaginous surfaces, allows for smooth motion. The cartilage covering the ends of the bones is made of a soft cushion-like material

123

that acts as a shock absorber and prevents the bones from rubbing against each other.

Arthritis is a progressive degeneration of the cartilage resulting from the wear and tear on the joint combined with the body's inability to regenerate the cartilage at the same pace. In an arthritic joint there may either be insufficient synovial fluid, causing stiffness, or an excess, causing swelling. If the cartilage has broken down enough to allow the bones to rub against each other, there is significant pain. The body often attempts to repair the joint damage by producing bony outgrowths at the margins of the affected joints. These spurs can also cause pain and stiffness.

The primary symptoms of arthritis are:

- Intermittent pain with motion of affected joints
- Stiffness and limitation of movement, with audible cracking in the joints
- Swelling and deformity of the joint
- Pattern of gradual onset

There are two types of osteoarthritis:

1. *Primary*—results from normal wear and tear
2. *Secondary*—results from an injury to a joint; from disease; or chronic trauma, such as obesity, postural problems, or occupational overuse

MEDICAL MARIJUANA RECOMMENDATIONS FOR OSTEOARTHRITIS

Since osteoarthritis is an inflammatory condition, the following recommendations are very similar to those in Chapter 5, with the exception of topicals for localized joint pain. These creams, sprays, and lotions can be highly effective for relieving pain without getting high, and are ideal for use while working during the day.

- Juicing raw cannabis leaves—for those without access to fresh plants, THCa tincture, CBDa tincture, and CBD tincture are excellent alternatives

- Topicals—localized (apply to painful joints): Apothecanna Extra Strength, Mary's Medicinals CBC
- Topicals—generalized (apply to wrist or ankle for rapid absorption) transdermal patches, especially 3:2/CBDa:THCa; THCa; 1:1/CBD:THC.
- Vaporize high-CBD strains of flower: Harlequin (a 50:50 hybrid), Lucy (a 70:30/I:S indica), Cannatonic (a 50:50 hybrid); other hybrids (either 50:50, 60:40/S:I or 60:40/I:S); or other high-CBD strains
- High-CBD tinctures: 1:1, 2:1, 3:1, 6:1, or 20:1/CBD:THC
- High-CBD hash oil: 3:1, 6:1, or 20:1/CBD:THC, either vaporized or ingested
- Indica strains of flower, with I:S of 70:30 or above
- Indica and hybrid edibles—gluten-free, without sugar or dairy
- Any strain or MMJ product containing CBG

NOTE: Use caution with sativa strains above 60:40/S:I and high-THC products. Although THC has anti-inflammatory properties and can be useful to some patients, it can also increase anxiety, which has the potential to increase inflammation.

HOLISTIC MEDICAL TREATMENT AND PREVENTION PROGRAM FOR OSTEOARTHRITIS

The most important time to start a holistic medical treatment plan is right at the onset of symptoms. If you start feeling abnormally stiff in the mornings, and are having some soreness in one or more joints, possibly accompanied by intermittent swelling, this is the critical time to start treating! If you act quickly you can prevent the joints from degenerating by reducing inflammation and saving the cartilage.

I've often seen patients who chose to live with the symptoms for many months or years and then suddenly their joints begin rapidly deteriorating. Pain becomes more severe, they're increasingly dependent on pain medication, mobility is more restricted, and they have joint replacement recommended by an orthopedist.

The HMTP Program can prevent this scenario. Even if you have been living with OA for several years, it's still possible to greatly improve and minimize further damage to your joints.

The three most important steps for preventing joints from degenerating and possibly reversing the early stages of damage are:

1. *Reduce inflammation*: Put a hose on the fire through the HMTP outlined below. This helps minimize damage to cartilage.
2. *Feed cartilage*: Cartilage does not have a direct blood supply, so you need to provide it with nutrients that are easily absorbed. This helps the cartilage repair, while keeping the synovial membranes healthy and the joints well lubricated.
3. *Exercise*: Keep the joint capsules healthy by proper exercise and conditioning. You want to exercise in a way that will not contribute to more joint wear and tear, so avoid any impact exercise, especially running or jumping. You might benefit from the guidance of a personal trainer or a physical therapist.

Risk Factors and Causes

- Genetic predisposition
- Severe or recurrent joint injury from heavy physical activity
- Skeletal postural defects and congenital joint instability
- Excess weight—excessive body weight and high body mass index are significant predictors of osteoarthritis of the knee. The risk for arthritis of the knee is 50 to 350 percent *greater* in men who are the heaviest compared to those of normal weight. This principle probably relates to other weight-bearing joints as well.
- Exercise—there is some evidence that only the most violent joint-pounding activities (long-distance running, basketball, etc.) performed over many years will predispose you to the development of arthritis.
- Cold climate and barometric pressure changes
- Food allergy, especially allergy to nightshades (potatoes, tomatoes, peppers, and eggplant), wheat/gluten, and dairy
- A diet high in animal products
- Low-grade infections, such as dental infections or infections in the gut that make the intestines "leaky," therefore adding to general toxic load and inflammation.

- Autoimmune disease
- Dehydration
- Excessive acid in the body causing increased amounts of calcium, minerals, and acid toxins to be deposited in the joint, resulting in inflammation and pain.
- Gut dysbiosis and leaky gut syndrome—recent research has shown that disordered gut bacteria (dysbiosis) may be creating toxins that increase inflammation throughout the body, in addition to leaky gut syndrome. This is a condition in which the gut lining becomes thin and damaged and begins to abnormally absorb toxins and incompletely digested food, which in turn, triggers joint inflammation. A holistic doctor can check for these problems with stool and blood testing and design an effective plan for reversing this causative factor.

Physical Health Recommendations for Reducing Inflammation, Feeding Cartilage, and Maintaining Joint Health

Arthritis, like any other chronic condition, is a systemic (whole body) dis-ease. It is not usually just a local dysfunction of a particular joint. If there is no major joint degeneration (i.e., you have no cartilage left—bone on bone), it is curable using a holistic whole-body approach.

Diet

The first step in treating arthritis is to *remove* all inflammatory causes. Many people with arthritis have food allergies that cause joint inflammation. Dairy products; wheat- and gluten-containing grains like rye, barley, and spelt; and (due to the acid they contain, called solanine) *nightshade plants*, which include potatoes, peppers, eggplant, tomatoes, and tobacco, are most often responsible for these food allergies. Eliminating all of them from your diet for at least one month (preferably for three months) will help to determine if a food allergy is contributing to your arthritis. You can then gradually reintroduce them (one food every three to four days) and carefully record, using the 0 to 10 pain scale, if you have a flare-up of joint pain. There is also now sophisticated food sensitivity blood testing that your holistic doctor can do to determine which foods you react to, and it can test up to 180 foods at a time.

The next step is to *remove* or decrease consumption of *all animal products* other than fish, which will help to eliminate excess calcium, mineral deposits, and acid from the joints. The most effective way to do this is to *eat a raw food vegetarian diet*. This is also called a vegan diet (vegetarian plus elimination of all animal products, especially dairy).

Even if you do this for only one to two months, there is an excellent chance that you will feel significantly better. If this is too extreme for you, then allow organic, chemical-free animal foods on a more limited basis, with a portion the size of the palm of your hand once or twice daily. Fresh wild-caught ocean fish, as well as eggs, chicken, turkey, and lamb are best if you are including animal protein. If you do nothing else, then strictly avoid dairy and red meat products.

The most effective way to dramatically reduce inflammation, increase joint comfort, and lessen stiffness is to do a supervised medical-grade detoxification program. There are a number of seven-, ten-, and twenty-eight-day professional programs based on good clinical and scientific research for rapidly reducing pain and inflammation.

Todd Nelson, a naturopathic doctor with whom I've worked closely for nearly thirty years (and a contributing author to this chapter), has guided several thousand people through these programs with exceptional results. Detoxification programs typically use Functional Medicine (a form of alternative medicine that focuses on interactions between the environment and the gastrointestinal, endocrine, and immune systems)–based food drinks along with low-allergy foods. If you are interested in these programs, Todd's contact information is available in Resources. He frequently guides patients long-distance via phone and Skype.

A more intensive approach to cleansing is periodic supervised *fasting*, which also has a very high success rate. This is not a new idea. For more than fifty years, fasting clinics throughout Europe have had outstanding results with periodic juice fasting. Gabriel Cousens, MD, at his Tree of Life Rejuvenation Center in Patagonia, Arizona, has administered to a number of people a juice fasting program for treating arthritis and has been consistently successful. Fasting enhances the eliminative and cleansing capacity of the lungs, skin, liver, and kidneys. It also rests and restores the digestive system and helps to relax the nervous system and mind. If you're considering fasting as a therapeutic option, it is best to do it under the supervision of a well-trained physician.

Refer to the anti-inflammatory diet in Chapter 5 for more specifics on reducing inflammation. Diet is a critical factor in slowing, or even stopping, the arthritic inflammation. There is no way to heal your joints without significant dietary changes.

Weight reduction, through diet and exercise, is also recommended in treating arthritis, as excess weight can accelerate joint deterioration.

Core Dietary Supplements

The following are professional dietary supplement recommendations we (Dr. Nelson and I) use in our clinics every day with great success. There are many supplements claiming to improve joint health and reduce inflammation, but the majority are not scientifically supported, have minimal quality control, and simply don't work. Each product suggested below is reinforced with substantial science and clinical data, along with the most stringent standards of quality control in the industry.

Wellness Essentials Active packets are formulated to feed cartilage, help your body to naturally reduce inflammation without the harsh side effects of anti-inflammatory medications, and promote general health. The result is improved joint flexibility, mobility, and comfort. This product is from Metagenics—see Resources.

The benefits the constituents of each packet provide (according to the manufacturer) are:

- *Multifaceted health support*: PhytoMulti is a high-quality multivitamin, containing essential nutrients and a proprietary blend of concentrated extracts and phytonutrients to help protect cells, maintain DNA stability, and activate health potential.
- *Pain relief*: Kaprex provides a safe option for effective joint pain relief, with a proprietary combination of selected plant components, particularly from hops.
- *Joint health support*: ChondroCare is a comprehensive formula designed to provide broad connective tissue support, with glucosamine, chondroitin, methylsulfonylmethane (MSM), and other nutrients.

- *Healthy cartilage support*: Glucosamine Sulfate 750 helps support healthy joints and other connective tissues by providing additional glucosamine, a naturally occurring compound in all connective tissues.
- *Anti-inflammation support*: OmegaGenics EPA-DHA 500 is a quality-guaranteed omega-3 fatty acid formula providing third party–tested omega-3 fatty acids to ensure greater purity.

Recommended dosage: Take one packet daily with food.

The primary nutrients included in the Wellness Essentials Active packets that are most effective for treating OA are the following:

- *Glucosamine sulfate*: Glucosamine is a naturally occurring chemical found in the human body, primarily in the fluid around joints. It can also be made in the laboratory and found in other places in nature. For example, the glucosamine sulfate that is put into dietary supplements is often harvested from the shells of shellfish. Glucosamine is a building block of cartilage and can be used to repair damaged or to grow new cartilage. Although it is not an anti-inflammatory, a multitude of studies (more than three hundred, including twenty double-blind studies) have shown that glucosamine can relieve the pain of osteoarthritis. This supplement is considered safe, but it can occasionally produce heartburn and diarrhea. It usually takes four to eight weeks to get significant benefit from glucosamine. If you are allergic to shellfish, you should not take this.
- *Chondroitin sulfate*: Chondroitin is a major component of cartilage that helps it retain water. It's extremely important to get high-quality, toxin-free chondroitin, which Wellness Essentials Active packets contain. Chondroitin taken with blood-thinning medications like NSAIDs may increase the risk of bleeding. If you are allergic to sulfonamides, start with a low dose of chondroitin sulfate and watch for any side effects. Other possible side effects include diarrhea, constipation, and abdominal pain.
- *Essential fatty acids*: There are many studies demonstrating the benefits of omega-3 oils from cold-water fish (salmon, sardines, and tuna) for people with OA. It's important to have extremely pure forms of fish oils that are not contaminated with heavy metals, cholesterol, or other

toxins. Organic *flaxseed oil* has also been shown to reduce arthritic inflammation. Take one to two tablespoons daily.

- *MSM*: MSM (methylsulfonylmethane) is frequently recommended for OA. There are many anecdotal reports of its benefit in treating the problem, but very little controlled data. MSM is hypothesized to deliver sulfur to arthritic joints, and thus act as an anti-inflammatory and pain reliever. MSM may also have a blood thinning effect. Be aware that MSM is not chemically related to sulfa drugs, and thus is not contra-indicated with sulfa allergy.
- *Kaprex*: hops extract. Metagenics is the only supplement company offering a joint health formula that is based on a patented hops extract that has been extensively researched for increasing joint comfort.

Additional Supplements

- *OmegaGenics SPM Active* (Metagenics): a fish-oil derivative that Harvard studies demonstrate accelerates the resolution of inflammation. Begin with a loading dose of two capsules three times a day with food for one to two weeks, followed by a maintenance dose of one to four capsules a day.
- *Vitamin D3*. See the recommendations for vitamin D in Chapter 5.
- *Niacinamide* is a B vitamin (B3), similar to niacin, which has been beneficial in treating arthritis. The recommended dosage is 500 mg three to four times daily, but some people will benefit with as little as 250 mg three times daily. The only reported negative side effect is that on rare occasions it can be harmful to the liver. A periodic liver profile (blood test) can monitor your liver function. Available in health food stores.
- *S-adenosyl methionine (SAM-e)* has been successful for treating arthritis for more than thirty years in Europe. You can try 400 mg one to two times daily. Found in health food stores.

Exercise

Yoga can be especially beneficial as part of the treatment program for arthritis. Whatever form of exercise you choose, it should not cause direct pounding or contribute to the deterioration of the affected joints. Swimming is a good choice for arthritis sufferers.

Professional Care Therapies

Traditional Chinese medicine, both acupuncture and Chinese herbs; Ayurvedic medicine, especially Boswellin Cream, camphor, and eucalyptus oil; bodywork (Rolfing and Hellerwork); body movement therapies, such as Feldenkrais, Trager, and Pilates (can improve mobility of the affected joints); chiropractic and osteopathic manipulation (can increase circulation to the joint); homeopathy; and craniosacral therapy can all be helpful in treating arthritis.

The Issues in Your Tissues

Louise Hay, in *You Can Heal Your Life*, lists as a probable emotional cause of arthritis: "Feeling unloved. Criticism, resentment." The affirmation that she recommends is: *I am love. I now choose to love and approve of myself. I see others with love.*

Caroline Myss, in *Anatomy of the Spirit*, writes that she believes the mental/emotional issues related to arthritis are:

- Sensitivity to criticism—probably the most significant emotional factor
- Trust
- Fear and intimidation
- Self-esteem, self-confidence, and self-respect
- Care of oneself and others
- Responsibility for making decisions
- Personal honor

There are a number of *affirmations* that you could create, directly related to the joints affected by arthritis or to the activity the arthritis prevents you from doing. For example: "My fingers move freely and easily." "My hands are filled with energy and vitality as I [write, type, work at my computer, paint, sculpt, play the piano]." Remember that you cannot use negative words. So you can't say, "I am [writing, painting, etc.] without pain." You could say, "My hands are free of pain," but that still focuses your attention to some extent on the pain. Try to make the affirmations as positive as possible.

In addition to writing and reciting the affirmations, you can also visualize and feel them (affirmations will be presented in more depth in Chapter 17). In addition to seeing your own affirmations, another effective *visualization* for arthritis would be to picture the surface of your arthritic joint as if it were healed. To do so, you could imagine the most perfectly smooth, grayish-white, glistening cartilaginous surface of a chicken or turkey drumstick that you've ever seen. Every day you could take a few minutes to picture in your mind's eye an irregular inflamed discolored cartilaginous surface being transformed into a perfectly healthy joint surface.

There is a published study that has documented the benefit of *journaling* about your feelings in treating arthritis (see Chapter 17).

RHEUMATOID ARTHRITIS (RA)

Less common and often more disabling than osteoarthritis, rheumatoid arthritis affects between 2 and 3 percent of the American population. Women are affected three times more than men. Although it most commonly occurs between the ages of thirty and forty, the disease can begin at any age. In childhood it is called juvenile onset rheumatoid arthritis and afflicts seventy-one thousand children every year—six times as many girls as boys.

Rheumatoid arthritis is chronic and progressive and is thought to be an autoimmune disease. These conditions occur when the body fails to recognize its own tissues or cells and initiates an immunological response in which antibodies attack parts of the joint tissue, as well as skin and muscles.

The joint damage caused by RA begins with an inflammation of the synovial membrane. This then leads to thickening of the membrane resulting from the overgrowth of synovial cells and an accumulation of white blood cells. The release of enzymes and other substances by these cells can erode the cartilage that lines the joints, as well as eroding the bones, tendons, and ligaments within the joint capsule. As the disease progresses, the production of excess fibrous tissue limits joint motion.

Since RA is a systemic disease, symptoms can affect the entire body.

Early in the course of the illness, even before the joints are involved, there can be fatigue and weakness, general feeling of malaise (feeling ill), low-grade fever, inflammation of the eyes, loss of appetite, and weight loss.

The disease can occur in many forms, from a mild short-term illness with little damage in only a few joints to a severe progressive condition with significant destruction of many joints. Most people are somewhere between these two extremes.

Joint symptoms include:

- Pain, swelling, and red/purple color of the finger joints (but not usually the joints closest to the fingertips), wrists, ankles, and toes—occurs symmetrically on both sides of the body (osteoarthritis does not present symmetrically)
- Warm and tender joints
- Stiffness, usually early morning, improves during the day
- Red, painless skin lumps called rheumatoid nodules, over the affected joints
- Bent and gnarled deformities (usually in fingers and hands) in long-term RA

There is no specific diagnostic test for RA, but from medical history, physical examination, joint X-rays, blood tests, and joint fluid analysis a definitive diagnosis can usually be made.

MEDICAL MARIJUANA RECOMMENDATIONS FOR RHEUMATOID ARTHRITIS

Like osteoarthritis, RA is an inflammatory condition. The MMJ recommendations are therefore much the same. However, the MMJ options are valued somewhat differently. For example, among the more than eighty cannabinoids, THCa is considered the most potent anti-inflammatory and is also effective in treating autoimmune conditions. THCa is not psychoactive and can therefore be used along with vaporizing a high-CBD hybrid, using a high-CBD tincture, or eating a high-CBD or hybrid edible. The topical creams, sprays, balms, and lotions can be highly effective for relieving pain without getting high. In conjunction with

THCa, they are ideal during working hours. THCa is available by itself in both a tincture and a transdermal patch. But perhaps the best choice for RA patients is to juice raw leaves for a strong analgesic combination of CBDa and THCa.

- Juicing raw cannabis leaves
- THCa—available in both tincture or transdermal patch; tincture is more effective since it closely parallels the THCa in raw cannabis juice. Recommend using it along with a high CBD:THC product.
- Topicals—localized (apply to painful joints)
- Topicals—generalized (apply to wrist or ankle for rapid absorption)-transdermal patches, especially 3:2/CBDa:THCa; THCa; 1:1/CBD:THC; and transdermal gel pens
- Vaporizing high-CBD strains of flower—Harlequin (a 50:50/S:I hybrid), Lucy (a 70:30/I:S indica), Cannatonic (a 50:50 hybrid); or other hybrids (either 50:50 or 60:40/S:I or 60:40/I:S)
- High-CBD tinctures—1:1, 2:1, 3:1, 6:1, or 20:1/CBD:THC
- Ingesting high-CBD hash oil—3:1 or 6:1/CBD:THC
- Indica strains of flower, with I:S of 70:30 or above
- Indica and hybrid edibles—gluten-free, without sugar or dairy
- Any strain or MMJ product containing CBG

NOTE: Avoid sativa strains above 60:40/S:I and high-THC products. Although THC has anti-inflammatory properties, it can also increase anxiety, which very often will increase pain.

HOLISTIC MEDICAL TREATMENT AND PREVENTION PROGRAM FOR RHEUMATOID ARTHRITIS

Risk Factors and Causes

As with all chronic conditions, there are multiple factors that predispose to the development of RA. Although the exact cause is unknown, there is strong evidence of a *genetic* component and an *immunological* problem. Evidence for the latter places RA in the category of an autoimmune disease (the body reacting against itself). Some researchers believe RA is triggered by either a *viral infection* or a *hormonal imbalance.* There is some evidence that the disorder is related to a distorted permeability of the small intestine. Others have identified *food allergies* and *psychosocial* factors as possible prime contributors to this condition.

Physical Health Recommendations

Although I am aware of some physicians who have observed significant improvement in patients using food elimination, there are very few well-documented cases of RA being successfully treated with holistic medicine. This may be a result of the advances made by conventional medicine in slowing the progression of the disease, coupled with the likelihood that many people with RA consult a holistic practitioner only during the latter, more disabling stages of their disease. The holistic treatment is most effective for milder cases of RA and is very similar to the approach used to treat osteoarthritis (see the preceding section), with the following exceptions and suggestions. *Early intervention is essential, before there is significant joint destruction.*

Diet

A *vegan* diet—vegetarian diet with all animal products, especially dairy and eggs, eliminated—is best. The exceptions to this diet are fish and high-DHA eggs (found in some health food stores). This diet can also serve as a food elimination diet to identify possible food allergens. The most highly allergenic foods associated with RA are dairy products, wheat/gluten grains, and corn. Some practitioners find *food sensitivities* significantly related to RA in up to *50 percent* of cases. (See the "Osteoarthritis" section for the remainder of the dietary suggestions.)

A twenty-eight-day cleansing program utilizing the product UltraInflamX Plus 360 from Metagenics can be very useful to rapidly reduce inflammation for people with RA, especially in the early onset of the disease. This must be done under the supervision of a Functional Medicine practitioner.

Vitamins, Minerals, and Supplements

The antioxidants, minerals, and supplements are essentially the same as for osteoarthritis, with the following *prioritized items*:

1. *Glucosamine sulfate*: not to the same extent as for osteoarthritis, but also considered moderately effective in treating RA; 500 mg three times daily.
2. *Vitamin C*: as ascorbate or Ester C; 1,000 mg three times daily
3. *Essential fatty acids*: especially EPA, an omega-3 (flaxseed oil is the most effective and economical means of taking it; daily dose is one to two tablespoons)
4. *Omegagenics SPM Active*: same dosage as osteoarthritis
5. *Copper*: 2 mg daily
6. *Quercetin or curcumin* (with bromelain): 250 mg between meals three times daily
7. *Manganese*: 30 mg daily
8. *Selenium*: 200 mcg daily

Digestive enzymes such as *pancreatin* have been helpful in treating RA, possibly by mitigating the effects of food allergies. The recommended dosage is 500 to 1000 mg with each meal. *Probiotics*, such as acidophilus- and bifidus-containing products, can help relieve the symptoms of RA by reducing bowel toxicity.

Herbs and Botanicals

- *Curcumin* (turmeric): the best-documented herb for treating RA; a potent anti-inflammatory, usually supplemented with any of the following products. I recommend Curcuplex (Xymogen), a highly absorbable curcumin extract. Dosage: one capsule three times a day before meals.
- *Bromelain*: a pineapple extract and enzyme that also acts as an anti-inflammatory
- *Bupleuri falcatum*: a Chinese herb that seems to be as effective an anti-inflammatory as steroids and without the harmful side effects; 2 to 4 gm daily
- *Siberian ginseng* (eleuthrococcus): a Korean herb that strengthens the adrenal glands; 500 mg two times daily
- *Hawthorn berries*: a rich source of flavonoids that helps to heal joint membranes; one-half teaspoon or two capsules three to four times daily

Professional Care Therapies

The same therapies used for treating osteoarthritis can be used for RA. Some holistic practitioners have had success in treating RA with bee venom therapy.

The Issues in Your Tissues

Certain personality traits tend to be associated with RA. Those at risk tend to be more compulsive, perfectionistic, overconscientious and helpful, excessively moralistic, and more frequently depressed. Many people suffering with this disease are rigid and stubborn, inflexible and immobile. In a survey of eighty-eight children with juvenile RA, the most striking findings were the psychosocial factors: children whose parents were unmarried comprised 29 percent, while adoption occurred three times more often in this population. The onset of the disease, in 51 percent of the cases, occurred very close to the traumatic event—divorce, separation, death, or adoption. RA sufferers of any age may have been more vulnerable to any instance of separation, either real or imagined. Once again, we clearly see evidence supporting the core belief of holistic medicine: *the perceived loss of love is our greatest health risk.*

In addition to the recommendations made for osteoarthritis, *psychotherapy* can be quite helpful for people suffering with RA. There are usually painful deep-seated emotional issues related to RA that need to be addressed and released before significant healing can occur. Enhancement of family support and family counseling are strongly recommended with RA. *Affirmations* and *visualizations* can also be of great value with this condition.

Patient Story—**Rheumatoid Arthritis**

Jessica R. is a thirty-five-year-old homemaker who homeschools her three young children. She was definitively diagnosed with RA in 2007, but she'd been having pain since age sixteen. Following her diagnosis, she was prescribed meloxicam, which she took briefly but stopped due to the severe abdominal pain it caused. Her only other medication was over-the-counter ibuprofen, which she took daily, often as much as 800 mg three times a day. It helped to somewhat relieve the severe pain she had in her hands, arms, shoulders, neck, knees, and ankles. But she was unable to exercise and her weight ballooned to 260 pounds.

She began taking MMJ in 2013 and experienced dramatic relief. After smoking a strong indica before bed, she was able to relieve her pain for nearly twenty-four hours. During the winter months her pain without MMJ was an 8, but it was reduced to a 2 with the indica or a 3:1/CBD:THC tincture; and during the summer months it dropped from a 5 to a 0 to a 1. She also uses the topical Apothecanna Extra Strength, which has helped tremendously with the pain in her hands. The MMJ has allowed her to sleep well, relieve her anxiety, and exercise on a regular basis, resulting in a weight loss of 120 pounds.

Patient Story—**Lupus Arthritis**

Nearly as common as RA is systemic lupus erythematosus (SLE), commonly known as *lupus*. SLE, like RA, is an autoimmune disease, a condition in which the body's immune system mistakenly attacks healthy tissue. The disease can affect the skin, joints, kidneys, brain, and other organs, but almost everyone with SLE has joint pain and swelling—i.e., *arthritis*.

Although I did not present SLE in this chapter, it is not an uncommon form of arthritis and this patient had a dramatic improvement with MMJ.

Twila Z. is a fifty-nine-year-old retired teacher who was diagnosed with lupus in 2007 shortly after developing symptoms of red patches and rashes on her chest and face area, fatigue, and swelling in her joints. She immediately began a course of steroids and Cytoxan (a chemotherapy drug). The side effects of the drugs were devastating. She became dizzy, fainted, and was taken by ambulance to the hospital with very erratic vital signs and a leg that had broken in three places.

The Cytoxan was stopped, and although that helped lessen the dizziness, she had two more falls in the next four years that caused repeat fractures in the same spots. The fractures were the result of weakened bones from the ongoing steroids. She was in a cast for three months, and was using assistive devices to get around, such as a walker, cane, and at times, a wheelchair.

She had to severely curtail her physical activity, due to the pain, swelling, and the fear of breaking a bone again. In 2012 she had to retire from teaching as a result of her physical limitations. "My weight ballooned and I was becoming a shut-in."

On the advice of her son, she applied for a medical marijuana license as an alternative to the drugs she was taking. The relief she obtained from CBDa patches and smoking cannabis was immediate, and through trial and error she has found what products work best for her. Her condition improved enough after a year of using cannabis products that she was able to have an ankle replacement done on a joint that had been broken three times in six years.

She still had to use assistive walking devices until 2016, to allow for complete healing of the surgery, but the pain was manageable, and gone completely for weeks at a time. Through the use of MMJ, she was able to endure a year of physical therapy, and is now able to walk one to three miles a day without any problems, and to work out thirty minutes daily on weight training.

"While cannabis cannot cure my lupus and cannot stop bad days where I am immobile, I have been able to stop the use of chemotherapy drugs and to cut back on my steroid use. The joy I feel doing basic things, like going to the grocery store without having to use a motorized cart, is immeasurable. I know that when the pain starts, a quarter of a CBDa patch will take away the pain in a half hour, and the patch won't weaken my bones, making them brittle. I may not be able to ice skate, ski, or do competitive swimming ever again, but I can travel and enjoy my day-to-day life; no tethers to having IV treatments getting in a plane or car.

"Medical cannabis has definitely made a huge difference in the quality of my life, and I am looking forward to the day when such treatment options are available worldwide, and not looked at with suspicion and fear. I am fifty-nine years old, and definitely not a "stoner." The myth of cannabis only being used for getting high is an antiquated fallacy; the more informed the population is about the successes of cannabis in the treatment of chronic pain and disease, the sooner that myth can be dispelled."

Chapter 7

Low Back Pain
Stretch Your Body and Mind

About 80 percent of all Americans will suffer from low back pain at some point in their lives. Backache becomes more common between the ages of thirty and fifty as the intervertebral disks lose some of their ability to absorb shock and backs become more unstable from inactivity and prolonged sitting. According to the National Center for Health Statistics, back pain is the fourth most common chronic ailment, the sixth most common reason for visiting an emergency room, and accounts for 13 million visits to primary care physicians' offices each year, making it one of the most common reasons for seeing a doctor. Back pain is responsible for 60 million lost working days each year, which in turn costs the economy $5.2 billion.

Although we often think of the back as a single entity, it is actually a complex connection of *bones*, *nerves*, *muscles*, and *ligaments* with multiple functions. Together, all these parts of the back allow us to do a variety of activities, to comfortably remain in one position, to balance ourselves, and to perform very complex movements. The nervous system also helps coordinate various motions so that the different muscles and joints in particular areas work together to allow for seamless movements and actions.

Backache is the term used to describe a variety of conditions. Since X-rays usually reveal no abnormality, your symptoms and a physical exam are the major components in establishing a diagnosis. However, up to 85 percent of patients with low back pain cannot be given a definitive diagnosis. The most common types of backache are:

1. *Sprain and strain*—often used interchangeably, the most prevalent forms of low back pain. A strain is usually an overstretched muscle, and a sprain a partially torn ligament, but in most cases of backache it isn't clear which one is the cause.
2. *Muscle spasm*—a painful, sustained, and involuntary contraction of muscles in the back.
3. *Disc problem (a slipped disc)*—accounts for only 2 to 4 percent of backaches. In actuality, the disc *herniates* or bulges from between two vertebrae and may eventually rupture. This bulging disc may push against a spinal nerve, causing shooting pains, tingling, or numbness to extend into the leg. Most often the affected spinal nerve is the sciatic, the largest one, and when that occurs the condition is called *sciatica*.

MRI (magnetic resonance imaging), considered the most high-tech diagnostic tool, is known to be inaccurate 10 to 20 percent of the time with backache. Yet thousands of painful and expensive surgical procedures are performed every year based on the results of MRIs that show slipped or herniated discs. This practice has continued despite a study published in the *New England Journal of Medicine* that found *no correlation* between structural abnormalities (e.g., herniated disc) revealed on MRIs and back pain.

MEDICAL MARIJUANA RECOMMENDATIONS FOR LOW BACK PAIN

Low back pain from all causes is the most common reason for using medical marijuana. People suffering with low back pain comprise a third of my MMJ patient population. The vast majority of these patients use MMJ on a daily basis, usually late afternoon, shortly after finishing their workday. They either vaporize or smoke an indica strain or ingest an indica edible. Remember that indica usually contains higher amounts of CBD (and lower THC content than sativa strains), which is not only a strong analgesic but reduces anxiety and is also an excellent muscle relaxant. The overall effect (with inhalation) is almost immediate pain relief and relaxation, just what most of us could use for an aching back following a stressful day at work.

Other effective MMJ options for backache:

- Topicals—localized (apply directly to painful area); this is especially helpful during work hours; not psychoactive and an effective analgesic for two to three hours
- Topicals—generalized (apply to wrist or ankle for rapid absorption)—transdermal patches, especially 1:1/CBD:THC and CBN (best used in the evening for pain and sleep)
- Vaporizing high-CBD strains of flower—especially Harlequin (a 50:50/S:I hybrid), Lucy (a 70:30/I:S indica), Cannatonic (a 50:50 hybrid); or other hybrids (either 50:50 or 60:40/S:I or 60:40/I:S)
- High-CBD tinctures—1:1, 2:1, 3:1, 6:1, or 20:1/CBD:THC
- High-CBD hash oil—3:1, 6:1, 12:1, or 20:1/CBD:THC
- Indica strains of flower, with I:S of 70:30 or above
- Indica and hybrid edibles—gluten-free, without sugar or dairy

If *sciatica* accompanies the backache, it is often a more severe pain and requires the strongest MMJ analgesic products, such as Harlequin, vaporized or in a tincture. THCa, a potent anti-inflammatory, is also helpful for sciatica, in either a tincture (preferred) or a transdermal patch. It can be used in conjunction with other MMJ products.

HOLISTIC MEDICAL TREATMENT AND PREVENTION PROGRAM FOR LOW BACK PAIN

Risk Factors and Causes

- Lifting heavy objects improperly—e.g., moving too quickly or awkwardly, or bending from the waist
- Poorly conditioned muscles (both back and abdominal) due to lack of exercise and flexibility and excessive exercise
- Posture problems and leg length discrepancy
- Prolonged standing, insufficient arch support, and inappropriate footwear, such as high heels
- Obesity and pregnancy
- Inadequate support from a soft mattress
- Uncomfortable workstations, such as chairs with improper support or working under an automobile or with heavy equipment

- Nutritional deficiencies, especially low protein, manganese, and magnesium intake (diuretics used to treat high blood pressure can lower magnesium), and constipation

Physical Health Recommendations

Yoga

From my own experience and that of several of my holistic medical colleagues, I believe that *yoga* may not only be the most therapeutic exercise, but is probably the single best self-care therapy for treating chronic low back pain. I've also been impressed by the survey results from the book *Backache Relief*, by Arthur Klein and Dava Sobel. Published in 1985, the survey asked people (they had 492 respondents) who had been treated for backache to evaluate their practitioners based on the extent of the relief they experienced following their treatment. Yoga instructors fared best, with 96 percent of the respondents experiencing moderate-to-dramatic relief from back pain after practicing the yoga positions they'd been taught. The complete results of the survey are as follows:

Practitioner	Moderate-to-Dramatic Temporary Relief (%)	Moderate-to-Dramatic Long-Term Relief (%)
Yoga Instructors	96	4
Physiatrists/Physical Medicine & Rehabilitation (PM&R)	86	0
Physical Therapists	65	8
Acupuncturists	36	32
Chiropractors	28	28
Osteopathic Physicians	28	15
Neurosurgeons	26	8
Orthopedists	23	9
Family Practitioners	20	14
Massage Therapists	10	63
Neurologists	4	4

Yoga (a Sanskrit word meaning *union*) is a Hindu spiritual and ascetic discipline. It refers to a balanced practice of physical exercise, breathing, and meditation to unify body, mind, and spirit, making yoga one of the most effective and ancient forms of holistic self-care. The benefits of this five-thousand-year-old system of mind-body training to improve flexibility, strength, and concentration are well documented. The basis of yoga is the breath, a variant of abdominal or belly breathing. There are a number of yogic systems. Hatha yoga is the best known in the West. Hatha yoga postures, or asanas, affect specific muscle groups and organs to impart physical strength and flexibility, as well as emotional and mental peace of mind.

There are a variety of hatha yoga forms available. Initially it is preferable to receive instruction for the first two or three months, due to the subtleties involved in yoga practice that are not apparent without firsthand experience of its practice under the guidance of a qualified yoga instructor.

While writing the book *Backache Survival* in 2002, I consulted with five yoga instructors and asked each of them, "What are your top three yoga asanas that you would recommend to someone with low back pain from any cause?" Wherever they overlapped, I added that pose to my list, and was able to compile my own list of what I consider the top ten yoga poses for treating low back pain. Each one is a relatively simple stretch that can be performed on a yoga mat or on a carpeted floor. In yoga there is no such thing as perfection or competition. It is not a goal-oriented practice, nor is there the belief "no pain, no gain." In fact, the beauty of yoga is that there should be *no pain*.

You should begin yoga or a daily stretching regimen only after you have given your back a chance to rest and heal following an injury or an acute flare-up of back pain. If you're someone with backache, the practice of yoga is too valuable for you not to at least give it a try. If practiced on a consistent basis, I've found it to be the most effective therapy for *long-term relief of low back pain*.

With all of the following poses listen to your body and stretch gently to the point of pain and then back off just enough so that you experience no pain. As you practice them daily, your flexibility will gradually increase, and you'll be able to stretch a bit farther without any pain. By trying to achieve too much too quickly you can slow your progress and possibly injure yourself. Hold each pose for five breaths or approximately thirty to sixty seconds while breathing abdominally and if possible through your nose. Unless specified otherwise, repeat each position twice. If a particular stretch is meant to be done on both sides of your body (e.g., the Knee-to-Chest should be done for both the left and right knee), then do each side twice. Commit to spending at least fifteen to twenty minutes daily practicing the following ten yoga poses. Remember to breathe. With some, you'll be instructed to coordinate your breath with the stretch (e.g., Cat-Cow). Yoga can be very relaxing as well as remarkably helpful for your aching back. Enjoy the process!

YOGA POSES FOR LOW BACK PAIN

Knee-to-Chest: This position gently stretches the muscles in the hips, buttocks, knees, hamstrings, and lower spine, and strengthens core abdominal muscles, while keeping the spine in a protected position. There are two options for performing this stretch. They both begin the same way. Lying on your back, slowly bring one knee up to your chest, or as high as you can without experiencing pain. You can keep your opposite knee bent or straight, whichever feels better (with back pain, it's usually more comfortable bent). In position **a**, clasp your hands on your shin between your knee and your ankle. In position **b**, clasp your hands on your lower thigh just above the back of the knee. In both positions, on every exhalation, gently pull or squeeze your knee closer to your chest. On every inhalation, relax. Keep the knee flexed with both the pulling/squeezing and releasing. Continue this slow rhythmical breathing, while squeezing and relaxing. Feel the stretching in your hip joint, knee, and lower back. Repeat the same sequence with the opposite knee.

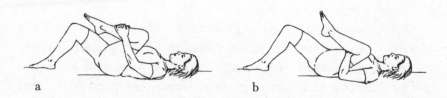

a   b

Supine Pelvic Tilt: Lie on your back with your arms to your sides and palms down. Bend both knees, keeping your feet flat on the floor. With each inhalation, arch your low back while keeping your hips on the floor (**a**). This will create a space between your low back and the floor. Exhale and press your low back into the floor (**b**). Repeat this movement of tilting your pelvis back and forth at least ten to twelve times.

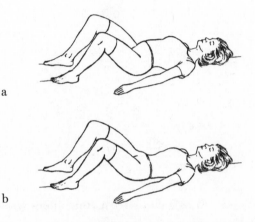

a

b

Cat-Cow: Turn over and place your hands directly under your shoulder joints, your knees under your hip joints, thighs and shins forming right angles. Your feet are in alignment with your knees. Toes point straight, and soles of feet face upward. Your spine has the same curves as it did when you were lying on your back in position b above, but now you are turned over, and with this movement your spine will flex and extend as you tilt your pelvis back and forth. Another benefit of this position is that because you are on your hands and knees, all of the weight is off your back, allowing for a greater capacity to stretch and heighten mobility of the spine.

For the Cat Pose (**a**), tuck your pelvis, drop your head, and round your back like an angry cat. Your hips (pelvis) are tucking and your spine is bending (flexing). This movement presses the air out of you, just like a bellows (exhale as you do it). You are also relaxing all the muscles in your head, neck, and shoulders as you do this stretch.

For the Cow Pose (**b**), tuck your pelvis as you inhale slowly, lift your head, look up, and gently release the arch from your thoracic spine (mid-back), forming a concave curve.

With both poses, move and breathe in a harmonious and relaxing rhythm while doing ten cycles initially and gradually working up to twenty-five cycles.

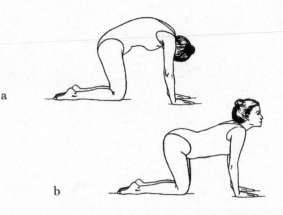

a

b

Chair Forward Bend: Sit in a chair with your knees wide apart, and your heels placed under your knees and your toes pointed slightly inward. Use a chair with a firm seat that allows your feet to be placed flat on the floor, or place books under your feet. Be sure your legs are parallel to each other, so that your shinbones provide support and you don't twist your knees. To begin, slide your buttocks to the back of the chair and tilt your trunk (from your waist up) forward to lean your elbows on your knees. Let your head hang forward so the back of your neck is stretched. If this position is too uncomfortable or if you have high blood pressure, glaucoma, or a detached retina, then maintain this pose for a few slow abdominal breaths and go no further. If none of these precautions apply to you, then tilt your trunk fully forward, letting your head and arms hang between your legs. If your hands don't touch the floor, then place them on books. Remain in this position and relax into it by tucking your chin slightly to stretch the back of your neck and soften the front of your neck as well. Hold this position for at least twenty to thirty seconds as long as you're not feeling pain. To come out of it, do not use your back muscles. Press your hands into the floor and begin moving up until your elbows rest on your knees, and then pause for several breaths. Then place your hands on your knees or on the seat of the chair, pushing your trunk upward while your head is still hanging forward. Straighten your head last, and then sit and breathe for another ten to twenty seconds without moving.

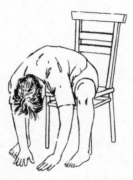

Cobra: Lie facedown on your belly. Place the palms of your hands on the floor in line with your chest and your fingertips in line with your shoulders, with your elbows close to your body, your feet together, and your forehead on the floor. Slowly extend your head so that your chin first touches the floor. Continue extending and lifting your head off the floor while raising your upper body. Use only your upper back muscles to lift (not your hands). Look up as you extend your head and neck as far as you can without straining, while feeling a backward bending in your spine. Come up only as high as is comfortable for you. Inhale as you do each progressive extension and raise your upper body. To lower, reverse the order, lowering your chest, then your chin, and then your forehead to the floor. Repeat this cycle five times. Remember to breathe and keep only light pressure on your palms so that your back muscles are doing the work. Try to relax the muscles in your buttocks as you maintain this position for as long as you can without forcing or straining. After completing at least five cycles, turn your head to one side, close your eyes, straighten and lower your arms to the floor, breathe, and relax. In addition to stretching and strengthening the muscles that extend your spine as well as your abdominal muscles, this stretch also helps to open up the disc spaces.

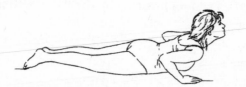

Desk Pose or Bridge: This pose is the counter pose of Cobra. Lie on your back and align your body as in the Supine Pelvic Tilt. This movement is very similar to the Cobra, except that now instead of your abdomen, your upper back becomes the base. Begin by exhaling and lifting your hips just an inch off the floor while keeping your waist-line on the floor. If it's not uncomfortable for you to do so, with each subsequent exhalation you can raise your pelvis higher, but do so very slowly (about an inch with each out breath). As you raise your pelvis, press down on your arms, hands, and the inside edges of the feet. Keep your knees and feet in alignment with the hip joints. Continue lifting up until you feel your lumbar spine (low back) beginning to arch.

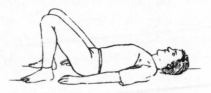

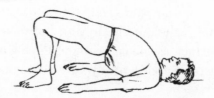

Hamstring Stretch: There are several methods for effectively stretching the hamstrings. Located in the back of the thigh, they are among the most powerful muscles in the body. Every yoga instructor with whom I consulted emphasized the importance of stretching the hamstrings in healing low back pain. (Surprisingly, it was the *only* one of these ten stretches selected as one of the top three by all five teachers.) I was given three hamstring options, which I'll present here.

(a) Lying on your back, bend one knee and bring it to your chest by clasping your hands behind your lower thigh just above the back of the knee. Then slowly straighten your leg at the knee joint, holding it in a vertical position, as close to ninety degrees as you can without forcing or straining. Hold the stretch for thirty to sixty seconds. It may be more comfortable to do this stretch if you bend the other knee while keeping that foot flat on the floor. To release this stretch you can slowly lower your leg to the floor, feeling its full weight as you lower it. Or if that's too uncomfortable, you can simply reverse the above stretch and bend your leg at the knee as you lower the leg and rest your foot on the floor. Repeat this stretch for the other leg.

(b) Begin this stretch just as you did in step a. However, instead of clasping your hands behind your thigh, place the center of a strap or belt on the ball of your foot before you gradually straighten your leg. Wrap the ends of the strap around your hands (ideally the strap should be six to eight feet in length) and hold for thirty to sixty seconds. The rest of this stretch is the same as step a.

(c) This hamstring stretch uses a doorway or a wall to support your leg, keeping your knee straight and stretching the hamstring. It's very similar to a and b, but with this one you can rest your arms on the floor. I find it a little easier to do than the other two and I'm able to hold the stretch much longer (two to three minutes). With all three of these options, remember to stretch both legs.

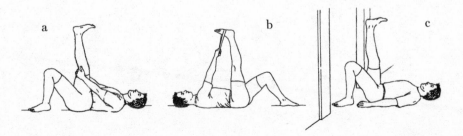

Forward Bend: Stand with your feet parallel, about hip width apart. Inhale while raising your arms up over your head with your palms facing each other. As you exhale, bend forward at the hips and gradually lower your hands toward the floor while slightly bending the knees (do not lock knees). Bend forward until you feel a gentle stretch in your hamstrings. Hold this position while breathing for thirty to sixty seconds.

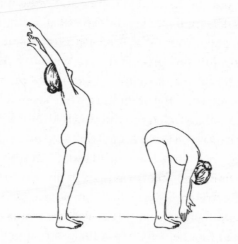

Easy Back Twist: Lie on your back with arms outstretched to the sides in a "T" position, with palms facing down. Bend your right knee and place your right foot on top of the left knee. Grasp your right knee with the left hand and gently draw the knee toward the floor on the left side of your body. Keep the right shoulder pressed to the floor, turn your head to the far right and gaze at your right hand. Hold for thirty to sixty seconds or five breaths. Release the knee and extend the leg and place it on the floor. Repeat the same sequence on the left side.

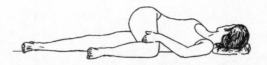

Relaxation Pose (Shivasana): This should be the final position of your yoga session. It will help you to become more fully relaxed, yet still conscious. It trains the body in stillness, the mind in alert quietness, and teaches systematic release of tension throughout the entire body. With each inhalation imagine that the breath is filling your chest, abdomen, back, and pelvis with cleansing or purifying air. With each exhalation, imagine that the breath is taking with it tension and toxins. Each in-breath can radiate in and illuminate every part of your body that it enters. It is helpful and can be especially healing to see a bright white light filling your low back with each breath. You should be very comfortable and warm in this pose, lying on a thick mat, a blanket (or under a blanket), or folded towels.

Begin by sitting on the floor with your knees bent and the soles of your feet on the floor. Place your hands behind your hips, palms down, with your fingers under your buttocks. Lean back on your elbows, your chin in, chest expanded, and shoulders away from your ears. Rest the back of your pelvis on your hands. Press your feet to the floor and gently push your body backward, hips sliding over hands, until your whole back, pelvis to shoulders, rests on the floor. Your head then comes to the floor with the chin tucked and neck elongated. Slide your hands out from under your hips and turn palms up. Extend your arms outward about fifteen degrees from your sides. Press your whole body downward into the floor—your feet, lower back, and the back of your neck and head. Feel your spine elongating. Exhale and relax. Extend first your right leg out on the floor, and then the left. Your feet, knees, and thighs turn outward. Now turn your attention to yourself, while trying to detach from any noise, activity, and your thoughts. You are aware of all of them but choosing not to give them any of your attention. Try to focus on your breath as it flows in and out, and feel the tension leave your body, from the crown of your head to the soles of your feet. Relax your tongue and your jaw muscles as your mouth opens slightly. Your arms and legs feel soft and heavy. Your hands and feet melt into the floor. Become very still and listen to the internal sounds of your body—the rhythmical beat of your heart, the breath flowing in and out. Use the imagery described above and rest in this relaxed state for about five minutes before you slowly come out of the pose. Begin to stretch your fingers and toes wide apart. Roll onto your side, knees to chest, hands cushioning your head. After a few breaths, come up to a sitting position. Sit for a few minutes with legs and ankles crossed, spine straight, head centered, and hands on knees. Feel gratitude for the healing gift you've just given yourself. In addition to the therapeutic benefit to your back, the consistent practice of yoga, even for just twenty minutes a day, is one of the most beneficial health practices I've ever experienced—for body, mind, and soul.

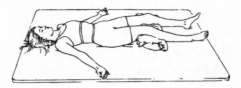

Bodywork and Body Movement

Maintaining the *structural alignment* of the muscles, tendons, joints, bones, and fascia (the lining of muscle) is an essential component of the holistic treatment for chronic low back pain. Several treatments by an osteopathic physician, chiropractor, or other trained or certified practitioner may be needed. Lasting benefit is most likely to be obtained with the more indirect types of treatments, such as *myofascial release* or *craniosacral osteopathy*. The more direct or high-velocity thrusting techniques, which force areas that are out of alignment back into alignment, are usually more helpful with acute injuries than with chronic back pain. However, other forms of *osteopathic* or *chiropractic* treatments, which usually consist of gentler techniques, can be helpful in some cases of chronic pain. But if these modalities or any other forms of therapy do not offer noticeable improvement after three to six treatments, it is important to evaluate whether to continue.

Physical therapy performed by a highly skilled therapist using a variety of modalities, such as heat, ice, ultrasound, and electrical stimulation, is often helpful. However, these are adjunct therapies and are not substitutes for structural treatment. They are unlikely to provide lasting relief with chronic pain when used alone. Standard physical therapy often utilizes strengthening exercises to overcome areas of weakness or misalignment. A holistic treatment program is designed to help the body to realign itself, thus healing the weakness and directly treating the cause of the problem.

There are several other forms of *bodywork* or *body movement therapies* that may be helpful in treating chronic low back pain. These therapies utilize methods to retrain the nervous system to improve posture, alignment, balance, coordination, and self-awareness. They can help you to move more efficiently and to be more aware of your body and how it works. Some of the more common body-based therapies include *Pilates*, *Feldenkrais*, *Rolfing*, and *Alexander Technique*. The *Lauren Berry Method* of bodywork is not as well known, but is also highly effective. These approaches often involve both hands-on treatments and instruction from the practitioner for exercises to be done by the patient at home. These exercises can directly address the cause of the back pain by helping the body to integrate its functions and resolve areas of dysfunction.

With any of these therapies for treating chronic back pain, you need to continually evaluate their benefit. If you are receiving the same treatment repeatedly without lasting results, the therapy is probably not addressing the underlying cause. Not only can continuing such a course of treatment become expensive, but it can also create a dependence on the practitioner. Holistic medicine attempts to address causes while empowering patients to learn to heal themselves.

Exercise

Yoga is the most effective exercise for both treating and preventing chronic low back pain. Remember—DON'T PUSH YOURSELF. If you keep it slow and steady, practicing every day, you might very well end up with a healthier back than you had prior to the onset of your back pain.

If you do not practice yoga, you should at least do several *stretching exercises* every day. A physical therapist can teach you, or you can refer to the book *Stretching* by Bob Anderson.

Brisk walking, swimming, or any other gentle form of *aerobic exercise* is recommended for treatment and prevention of chronic backache.

Acupuncture

Acupuncture may be helpful for both acute and chronic back pain. It may offer substantial and long-lasting relief, and it often works well in combination with structural approaches. The sooner the problem is addressed with acupuncture, the better the chance that it will work.

Sleep Support

Be sure your bed provides good support. Waterbeds and soft mattresses should be avoided.

Diet

Being overweight is a significant risk factor for chronic low back pain. If this applies to you, then I'd suggest following the candida-control, anti-inflammatory, hypoallergenic diet presented in Chapter 5. It's a highly nutritious, low carbohydrate diet that nearly always results in significant weight loss.

Bioenergy Recommendations

Energy medicine, using Healing Touch or Reiki, can be helpful in treating chronic low back pain. They work similarly to acupuncture, but instead of the specific meridians used by acupuncturists, these modalities should be applied directly to the low back. Using imagery while being treated by a practitioner of energy medicine will often enhance the effectiveness of the treatment.

The Issues in Your Tissues

Fear is the underlying emotion contributing to backache. Louise Hay, in her classic book *You Can Heal Your Life*, writes that a *fear of money and lack of financial support* may contribute to backache. People with low back pain also tend to have a *need for control*, so part of their stress may be a fear of being out of control or losing control.

Sciatica is often associated with *concerns about financial security*.

Caroline Myss, in *Anatomy of the Spirit*, believes the mental/emotional issues that may be associated with low back pain are those of the first and second chakras (the energy centers described in Ayurveda, the traditional medicine of India). These *issues in the tissues* of the low back are:

- Family relationships and group safety and security
- Ability to provide for life's necessities
- Ability to stand up for self
- Comfortably occupying one's home
- Social and familial law and order
- Blame and guilt
- Money and sex
- Power and control
- Creativity
- Ethics and honor in relationships

Louise Hay believes that backs represent the support of life and suggests the following affirmation for preventing back pain: *I know that life always supports me.* Specifically for low back pain, she suggests: "*I trust the process of life. All I need is always taken care of. I am safe.*"

Just as with any other malfunctioning part of the body, there are a wide variety of affirmations that you can create that will represent a healthy back to you. Some examples might be: *My back is strong and flexible. I am sitting, standing, bending, and lifting normally. My back is now completely healed. I am stretching every day and my back continues to heal.*

Relaxation techniques and *biofeedback* work well for backache related to muscle spasm and muscle tightness—the variety of backache often related to chronic stress.

Visualizations that represent healing are very powerful. Whatever your understanding of the cause of your back pain, it can be used to create a healing image. If the cause of your pain is unknown, then just ask for a healing image to come to you and use it every day while doing a breathing exercise. You could imagine each breath filling your abdomen and low back with light and energy, or a laser beam of light zeroing in on any abnormal tissue or contracted muscle. The light could either heal the tissue or relax the muscle enough to allow for a realignment of the spine to take place. Since the regular practice of visualization has been known to successfully dissolve cancerous tumors, it can certainly help to relax tight muscles and move bones.

Counseling can also be helpful in treating chronic low back pain.

Patient Story—**Low Back Pain**

The following story is a dramatic but typical account of the many positive treatment outcomes I've seen using medical marijuana for chronic low back pain.

Bruce S. is a forty-three-year-old computer programmer in Boulder, married, and the father of two, with a passion for the outdoors. A day after he slipped and fell on a rock while hiking with his family, he awoke with back pain so severe that he was unable to get out of bed. Muscle spasms seized his back with the slightest movement. A searing sciatic pain, radiating down to his knee, left him almost totally incapacitated.

Bruce's physician referred him to an orthopedic doctor, who, following an MRI revealing a partially ruptured disc in his lumbar spine, immediately recommended surgery. Bruce and his wife did some quick research and found that back surgery generally has a low success rate, so they decided to explore other treatment options. He visited a chiropractor, physical therapist, massage therapist, and an acupuncturist, but their treatment provided only minimal, temporary pain relief. His doctor prescribed various narcotics, primarily oxycodone, which masked the pain for a few hours, but he hated the side effects: drowsiness, constipation, and nausea.

After a few weeks, Bruce couldn't live with the pain any longer, so he decided on surgery. His fears were confirmed: the surgery didn't work. There was minimal improvement for the first few weeks, but he still continued with daily doses of oxycodone just to function. After several months he saw a pain medicine specialist who told Bruce that he should consider another surgery. More drugs, including antidepressants and muscle relaxants, were prescribed. Now a chronic condition, Bruce's back pain was straining his marriage; he could no longer sit on the floor with his baby daughter or lift his toddler son.

After more than a year of dead-end treatments, Bruce limped into my office in Boulder. Not only was his back pain excruciating, but also the ordeal had left him suffering severe bouts of anxiety and depression. Bruce felt hopeless and desperate. He admitted to being addicted to oxycodone.

"I have no life," Bruce said. "I can't even play with my kids. I'm not sleeping, and I'm concerned about losing my job."

Bruce was an ideal candidate for medical marijuana—specifically the indica strains that are typically high in CBD. In addition to marijuana, I suggested a regimen for gradually tapering off oxycodone. I also recommended daily yoga and gentle stretching, as well as a program of mindfulness and self-reflection.

After six weeks of daily doses of medical marijuana, Bruce returned to my office a different person, physically and emotionally. He had reduced by half his daily dosage of the narcotic pain relievers. After three months, he had stopped the drugs completely, relying solely on medical marijuana for pain relief, and continued with the holistic program of yoga and meditation. He and his wife were getting along better, his boss was pleased with Bruce at work, he was sleeping through the night, and he was lifting and playing with his children.

Chapter 8

Migraine Headache
Practice Self-Compassion

> *Cannabis is probably the most satisfactory remedy for migraine.*
>
> —Sir William Osler, MD, one of the founding
> professors of Johns Hopkins Medical School
> and revered by today's medical community
> (1849–1914; this statement from the late 1890s)

Migraines are the most common presentation of what are known as vascular headaches, a category that also includes cluster headaches. They are thought by most authorities to occur as a result of a spasm (constricting/narrowing) in the arteries at the base of the brain, triggering the visual "aura," followed by rather sudden relaxation and dilation of the same arteries that trigger the phase of throbbing pain. Blood flow to the brain during the early vasoconstrictive phase of a migraine episode is severely compromised, so much so that ministroke-like effects are occasionally seen as a residual.

The Migraine Research Foundation reports that 18 percent of American women suffer from migraines and 6 percent of men, approximately 38 million people. Though more difficult to diagnose because the presenting symptoms are more obscure, migraine does also occur in children.

The classic migraine headache is one-sided and is frequently heralded by the onset of an *aura* of visual disturbances consisting of bright spots, zigzag lines, blind spots, or temporary loss of part of the visual field on the side involved. The pain is often severe and incapacitating. Untreated, the throbbing or pounding pain can last for hours or days and is often severe enough to also induce nausea and vomiting. It is often accompanied by excruciating sensitivity to light that forces the sufferer to seek shelter in a darkened room. Typical age of onset is before age thirty-five. The symptoms in children tend to be nonspecific, with nausea, malaise, vertigo, and abdominal pain being more common than the headache itself. Migraine episodes recede with advancing age, and postmenopausal women have a much lower incidence.

MEDICAL MARIJUANA RECOMMENDATIONS FOR MIGRAINE HEADACHE

In a study done at the Skaggs School of Pharmacy and Pharmaceutical Sciences at the University of California, San Diego, researchers found inhaled and ingested cannabis to decrease symptoms of migraine. The study's sample was 121 adults, of which 40 percent reported positive effects following the consuming of cannabis. Additionally, about 85 percent of participants reported having fewer migraines per month with cannabis. Participants found that inhaled cannabis reduced migraine symptoms faster than ingested cannabis.

Cannabis in tinctures was the most effective treatment for migraine in the U.S. through the latter half of the nineteenth and the early twentieth centuries, until marijuana was declared illegal in 1937.

Smoking or preferably vaporizing high-sativa flower strains or high-THC hash oil is typically recommended for treating migraine headaches. *Timing* is critical, and MMJ should be inhaled as soon as the aura of an impending migraine headache begins or within twenty minutes of the onset of the aura (or the earliest symptom that lets you know a migraine is imminent). The majority of migraine sufferers report that a "full-blown" migraine typically occurs within twenty to forty minutes of the beginning of the aura. As soon as you're certain that a migraine is on its way (whatever the symptom is), that's the best time to vaporize.

At the present time smoking and vaporizing are the most dependable delivery methods that work quickly enough to knock out the migraine before the pain becomes intolerable. However, since smoke is a possible trigger for migraine headaches, vaporizers are preferred over smoking. Although sativa strains typically contain higher amounts of THC, when they're used for treating a migraine the psychoactive effect of the THC is not nearly as evident as if the same strain were used without a migraine.

I've also heard from a few patients with migraine headaches that if they are unable to vaporize flower during the initial window between the early warning and the onset of pain, and they're left with intractable disabling pain, dabbing concentrates can relieve it. Once a migraine begins, this seems to be the only method of delivering marijuana capable of significantly reducing the pain.

As mentioned in Chapter 3, THC is a central vasodilator, which means that it dilates arteries to the brain, heart, and kidneys. This effect makes THC the ideal antidote for the vasoconstriction of the arteries to the brain that causes the aura. We can only speculate, but it makes good physiologic sense, that if THC relieves the constriction of these arteries to the brain, then they most likely will return to their normal size and are *not* dilated from the THC, as they would have been had an aura not been occurring. This is probably the reason that you don't get as high from a sativa if you've used it to treat a migraine.

Perhaps the most effective strain for quickly preventing a migraine, if used at the appropriate time, is Durban Poison, a 70:30/sativa:indica. However, since stress/anxiety is the primary trigger for migraine headaches, and THC can potentially increase anxiety, I would also try using a 50:50 hybrid or a 60:40 sativa-dominant hybrid, and see if that works. Many patients report that these hybrids are often just as effective for treating migraines as the stronger sativas.

It's also important to note that nearly all of my migraine patients have been able to stop taking their prescription medication, which is most often Imitrex (sumatriptan), after they begin using MMJ. And they're very happy to do so, since Imitrex may cause several unpleasant side effects, such as dizziness, nausea, vomiting, and drowsiness. As with many of the pharmaceuticals, it relieves the pain but may render you unable to function normally.

Other MMJ options for *treating* migraines:

- Apothecanna Extra Strength or Mary's Medicinals THC-sativa cream—a localized topical; effective if applied during the window between the aura and the onset of the headache, to both temples and forehead between the eyebrows. It should begin to have an effect within five minutes.
- Sativa tinctures—can potentially minimize the headache if they start working within thirty minutes from the beginning of the aura. Most tinctures take at least thirty, and often forty-five, minutes to begin working. This means you should have the tincture with you at all times, so you can take it immediately with the onset of the aura. Tinctures seem to work more quickly with an empty stomach, in addition to holding them under your tongue for ten to fifteen minutes, or even longer.
- Sativa MED-a-mints sublingual tablets—relatively new and haven't been tested enough to recommend with certainty, but they do have the potential to begin working within twenty to twenty-five minutes if you adhere to the suggestions above for tinctures.

I've seen many migraine patients who report that their daily (or almost daily) use of MMJ has considerably reduced both the frequency and intensity of their headaches. If MMJ is used daily as a preventative measure, your primary objective is to reduce anxiety and stress.

MMJ recommendations for *preventing* migraines:

- Avoid sativa-dominant strains of flower and *vaporize* (no smoking) only 50:50 hybrids or indica-dominant hybrids.
- Use indica or high-CBD *tinctures* and *edibles*.
- Use CBD-only capsules.

HOLISTIC MEDICAL TREATMENT AND
PREVENTION PROGRAM FOR MIGRAINE HEADACHE

Risk Factors and Causes

Migraines can be caused or triggered by:

- Genetic predisposition—positive family history, in about one-half of people who experience migraines. There is considerable evidence that migraine-prone persons have low baseline levels of serotonin.
- Food sensitivities—see Headache Relief Diet below. Approximately one-half of all migraineurs (migraine sufferers) have a sensitivity/allergy to a food or beverage that triggers a headache.
- Histamine-containing and -releasing foods
- Chemicals (nitrates, monosodium glutamate [MSG], nitroglycerin, aspartame)
- Blood levels of magnesium well below levels in healthy people (predisposes to greater arterial constriction)
- Withdrawal from caffeine (caffeine constricts arteries)
- Smoke
- Sleep problems (too little or too much)
- Fatigue and exhaustion
- Weather changes, barometric changes, sun exposure
- Sun glare (off snow and water) and eyestrain
- Rebound from withdrawal of analgesic or vasodilating drugs
- Stress. A classic story is the onset of the headache in the let-down period immediately after an acutely stressful episode has passed. Numerous papers have described the precipitation of headache in migraine sufferers by submission to a stressful interview in which the patient has little control.
- Emotional changes and intense emotional experience. Anxiety and depression are strongly related to vascular headaches of both cluster and migraine varieties. Astute observers and researchers of migraine think there is a strong association with intense organized activity to attempt to manage feelings of anxiety, which drives the sympathetic nervous system to extremely high activity.

- Hormonal changes—menstruation, ovulation, oral contraceptives. Migraines are more common before and during a menstrual period and in women who take oral contraceptives. They are less common in pregnancy and in postmenopausal women. In migraine-prone pregnant women, headaches are much more common if pre-eclampsia is present; both conditions are related to lower levels of magnesium and are also often related to subnormal levels of progesterone.
- Chronic candidiasis—there is a higher percentage of migraine patients with high positive candida antigen or antibody titers than in a normal population. A majority of these migraineurs enjoy marked improvement or cessation of migraines when the yeast infection is treated.

Physical Health Recommendations

Headache-Relief Diet—Foods to Avoid

I. Foods High in Tyramine (an amino acid that can trigger migraines)

- *Ripened cheeses*
  Blue, Boursault, brick (natural), Brie, Camembert, cheddar, Emmentaler, Gruyère, mozzarella, Parmesan, Romano, Roquefort, Stilton; permissible cheeses are: American, Velveeta, cottage cheese, and cream cheese
- *Aged meat and fish*
  Liver, caviar, pickled herring, fermented sausage (bologna, pepperoni, salami, summer sausage), and processed meats (hot dogs and ham)
- *Alcoholic beverages*
  Red wine (chianti in particular), beer, sherry
- *Vegetables*
  Sauerkraut, pods of broad beans (string, lima, pinto, garbanzo, and navy beans; and peas)
- *Fruits*
  Avocados (especially if overripe—i.e., guacamole), bananas (especially if overripe), figs (especially canned), citrus fruit (no more than one serving per day: one orange or grapefruit, or one glass of orange juice), papayas, raisins

- *Any fermented, pickled, or marinated food*
  Vinegar (especially red wine vinegar), yogurt, sour cream, buttermilk, soy, yeast extracts, brewer's yeast, and sourdough bread

II. Foods That Dilate the Blood Vessels and Therefore Can Precipitate a Vascular Headache

- *All alcoholic beverages*
  If you must drink, the following are recommended: Seagram's V.O., Cutty Sark, Haute Sauterne Riesling, vodka (these are all low in tyramine).
- *Monosodium glutamate* (MSG)
  May be identified on food labels as hydrolyzed vegetable protein, natural flavoring, or seasoning. Found in Chinese foods, canned soups, frozen dinners, Accent, Lawry's Seasoning Salt, Hamburger Helper, etc. Check labels of all canned and packaged foods, as well as chips and other snack foods, many of which contain MSG.
- *NutraSweet (aspartame) and AminoSweet*
- *Nitrites*
  Hot dogs, turkey dogs, chicken dogs, bacon
- *Excessive amounts of niacin (niacinamide is fine) and vitamin A (over 25,000 IU daily)*

III. Other Foods That Can Cause Headaches

- Cow's milk, gluten grains (wheat, rye, barley, and spelt), corn, oranges, eggs, beef, yeast, chocolate, cane sugar, mushrooms, nuts, and seeds (sunflower, sesame, pumpkin)
- Caffeine, from coffee, cola drinks, and nonherbal teas (no more than two cups per day); and some aspirin medications, such as Anacin, Excedrin, and Vanquish—check the labels.
- Raw garlic and onions (cooked are fine)
- Hot fresh breads, raised coffee cakes, and raised doughnuts

IV. Eat Regularly, Don't Skip Meals

This may result in hypoglycemia, which is another headache trigger.

Other Dietary Recommendations

Nutritional recommendations for prevention of migraine include *decreasing fats* from land animals and *increasing foods* that inhibit platelet aggregation (stickiness), including vegetable oils, onion, garlic, and fish oils. I recommend the Fully Alive Diet (see Chapter 5).

- Food elimination: In a number of studies of foods and migraine, a majority of migraine sufferers improved on elimination diets. This means eliminating all suspected food allergens and then challenging your system by adding one food back in at a time, waiting two to four days, and noting if you get a headache. This is an accurate way to determine specific food offenders that you should now avoid.

- **Vitamins, minerals, and supplements:**

  1. Since *magnesium*-deficient people are more subject to migraine headache, adequate intake (400 to 600 mg/day) from food or supplements is essential. I recommend a powder that combines magnesium-L-threonate with magnesium glycinate for best effect. Both of these types of magnesium are very well absorbed, easily tolerated by the gut, and have been shown to reduce the frequency of migraines. The powder is called OptiMag Neuro from Xymogen. Take two scoops in water in the evening or before bed. This can be extremely effective.

     Intravenous injection of one to two grams of magnesium by your physician can terminate an *acute migraine* headache within minutes—in up to nearly 100 percent of subjects in some reviews. Intravenous injection of *folic acid*, 15 mg, in one study achieved total subsidence of acute headache within one hour in 60 percent, with great improvement in another 30 percent. These two agents are strikingly successful.

  2. *Omega-3 oils* (EPA and DHA, average dose 1,400 mg daily) greatly reduce intensity and frequency of migraines. I recommend Omega-Genics EPA-DHA 720 (Metagenics): one capsule two to three times a day.

3. *Vitamin B2* (riboflavin) 400 mg daily for three months has been shown to reduce migraine frequency by two-thirds.

4. *Vitamin C* (2,000 mg/day)

5. *Vitamin E* (400 to 600 IU/day)

6. *Vitamin B6* (100 mg/day)

7. *Choline* (100 to 300 mg/day); all of these vitamins plus choline reduce the tendency toward high platelets in migraine.

8. *5-hydroxytryptophan* (5-HTP) (300 mg two times a day) works well for prevention of migraine, enhanced by taking with 25 mg of vitamin B6. This works by increasing serotonin, which is usually low in migraine sufferers. Do *not* take this if you are currently taking Imitrex.

• Herbs

1. *Butterbur extract*, 75 mg daily of a pyrrolizidine alkaloids–free (PA-free) extract. This can be used preventively. For the past three years I have been recommending to my migraine patients a supplement called *Butterbur Extra* (see Resources), which in addition to butterbur, contains magnesium, vitamin B2, and feverfew. For the vast majority of the patients who have taken it on a daily basis, it has been highly effective for reducing both the frequency and intensity of migraine.

2. *Feverfew* (*Tanacetum parthenium*), 0.25 to 0.5 parthenolide content daily, has markedly helpful effects in migraine.

3. *Dried ginger*, 500 mg four times daily, and pueraria root also provide substantial benefit with reduction in frequency and intensity of migraine occurrences.

• Hormones: *Natural progesterone.* Some women can be prone to migraines pre-period, and can experience great relief by using *natural progesterone* during the last two weeks of their menstrual cycle. This should be done under supervision of a holistic physician.

Exercise

Brisk walking, jogging, sports activities, gardening, low-impact aerobics, and water aerobics are among the options for appropriate regular *aerobic exercise* that both releases tension from the system and reduces the frequency and intensity of migraine episodes.

Professional Care Therapies

Acupuncture in skilled hands can be very effective in treating migraine headache. In one study 40 percent of patients achieved a 50 to 100 percent reduction in severity and frequency of migraine episodes during treatment with acupuncture. Among the points that can also be conveniently used for *acupressure* are the following:

- The Hoku point in the soft tissue between the thumb and index finger
- The B2 point below the inner aspect of the eyebrow
- The GB20 and GV16 points over the spine and on both sides of the spine just below the back of the skull

The Issues in Your Tissues

Since 2011, I have seen more than six hundred patients who are using MMJ to treat and prevent their migraine headaches. The vast majority have been successful in significantly reducing the pain and frequency of their headaches. However, what I find most remarkable is the personality trait that nearly *every one of them* shares. People with migraine are very *hard on themselves*, and many will acknowledge, "You're not the first person who's told me that." They tend to be perfectionists and hold themselves to a very high standard of performance, and it doesn't seem to matter what the activity is that they're engaged in. They could be cleaning their own house, working as a senior executive, performing as a professional athlete—and it's not a boss, teacher, spouse, or parent telling them what to do. They do not have to meet someone else's expectations. Their pressure is *self-imposed*. This mind-body connection is fascinating, and most migraine patients are shocked at how well I seem to know them, in spite of the fact that we're meeting for the first time.

I've also learned from a medical intuitive that people with migraines have this belief: *I am not smart enough.* This belief might be the source of their perfectionism.

The most emotionally healing recommendation for migraine patients is the daily *practice of self-compassion.* Many people with migraine feel trapped by their circumstances and the gulf between the way life is and the way it *should* be. Releasing the demands (the "shoulds") with a strong dose of forgiveness can lead to rewarding and sometimes dramatic changes. To practice self-forgiveness on a regular basis, I suggest the affirmation *I'm always doing the best I can,* and its corollary *There are no mistakes, only lessons.*

Biofeedback and Relaxation

Learning and regularly practicing *biofeedback* or any of the systematic relaxation approaches achieves a *50 to 80 percent reduction or elimination* in both severity and frequency of migraine headache. You can achieve the same results by learning and practicing regular *meditation*, which will help you eliminate or reduce your need for medication. *Hypnosis* too has significant success with migraine. Self-hypnosis has been shown to be particularly helpful in children and teenagers.

Patient Stories—Migraine

Jason P. is a forty-two-year-old IT manager who has been getting migraines since the age of five. Prior to moving to Colorado, he lived in Texas where he was prescribed a number of medications (including Imitrex), none of which was effective. Over-the-counter ibuprofen worked best but still didn't prevent him from being temporarily incapacitated while he was working. He'd have to turn off the lights in his office and lie down on the floor for an hour or more before resuming work in a somewhat compromised state, still dealing with the headache.

I first saw him shortly after he moved to Colorado, and I recommended MMJ. At that time the migraines were occurring at least once a week, always triggered by stress. He did not have auras; his first warning of an impending migraine was a tension headache that usually began in the back of his neck at the base of his skull. I instructed him to vaporize a sativa as soon as possible after the tension headache began, and this proved highly effective for preventing the onset of the migraine.

I recently saw Jason for his fourth annual renewal of his MMJ license. The migraines are no longer a significant problem for him. They occur approximately once a month, but are never incapacitating. He's able to prevent them by vaporizing a sativa, usually Durban Poison (a 70:30/S:I strain), as soon as he feels the headache starting.

On this last office visit, Jason mentioned a significant change he's made. He now vaporizes an indica on a daily basis after work. This not only helps him relax, but also the mild psychoactive effect has given him more clarity on how self-critical he is (he was raised by a highly critical mother), and "it helps me to not be so hard on myself." He frequently repeats (to himself) the affirmation *I'm always doing the best I can*, and overall he believes this is helping him also to be a better and more forgiving parent for his three young children.

Debbie P. is a thirty-three-year-old chemist working for a pharmaceutical company and is currently engaged in developing an anticancer drug. She's been plagued with migraine headaches since age fifteen, and until she began using MMJ, about four years ago, she'd been taking Imitrex (Sumatriptan) to relieve the migraines.

At that time, her headaches occurred two to three times a week, usually late afternoon, toward the end of her workday, and almost never on the weekends. They were incapacitating. She would have to leave work immediately and take an Imitrex. The drug made her too drowsy and the pain was too debilitating to continue working.

After her first visit in 2012, I suggested Debbie take Butterbur Extra on a daily basis, which she did for about six months. This reduced both the frequency and intensity of the headaches. At the same time I also recommended that she repeat the affirmation *I'm always doing the best I can*, whenever she heard her inner critic questioning a decision or telling her she'd made a mistake. In addition, during this time frame, she often vaporized an indica to relax after work.

At the present time, she's getting migraines once or twice a month and treats them with either vaporizing a sativa strain (60:40 or 70:30/S:I) or, when that's not possible, applying the topical Apothecanna Extra Strength, which she always keeps in her purse, to her temples. Sometimes she will use both methods. The topical is not as effective as vaporizing the sativa, but it does relieve the pain, and now she rarely has an incapacitating headache requiring her to leave work early.

She acknowledges that although she sometimes falls back on old behaviors, she's not nearly as hard on herself as she used to be, and finds it easier to relax. Her headaches are vastly improved and she hasn't taken an Imitrex in more than three years.

Chapter 9

Fibromyalgia
You Are Your Highest Priority

Fibromyalgia (FM) is a mysteriously debilitating syndrome that afflicts between 6 and 12 million people in the United States. The condition bears a striking resemblance to chronic fatigue syndrome and affects mostly women (female to male ratio is about 10:1) between the ages of twenty-five and fifty. It is estimated that 15 to 20 percent of patients seen by rheumatologists have FM. Health care costs for people afflicted with this condition average about $10,000 per year, and FM patients are almost six times more likely than the general public to apply for disability payments. More than 25 percent of FM patients who remain employed report missing more than 120 days of work per year due to their disease.

The primary symptoms of fibromyalgia are generalized *muscle pain*, *muscle tenderness*, *stiffness*, and *aching*, along with significant *fatigue*. Other symptoms include sleep disorders, depression, poor memory and concentration, headache (tension or migraine), dizziness, tingling of the extremities, irritable bowel syndrome, irritable bladder (urgency and frequency of urination), temporomandibular joint syndrome (TMJ), cold intolerance, and allergic reactions to drugs, chemicals, and environmental toxins. Blood tests and X-rays normally do not reveal any specific abnormality. Ruling out rheumatoid arthritis, lupus, and other conditions with similar symptoms (especially pain and fatigue) to FM is an important part of the diagnostic evaluation. Some physicians believe FM to be a variant of chronic fatigue syndrome, since 90 percent of patients with FM report significant fatigue.

After many years of research, there is still no effective conventional medical treatment for fibromyalgia. Lyrica, an anticonvulsant, is often prescribed for FM pain. However, it can cause drowsiness, dizziness, dry mouth, constipation, and blurred vision. Antidepressants, such as Cymbalta, have been used to provide short-term relief for sleep disorders and depression, while anti-inflammatory medications have been used for treating the pain, with poor to fair results.

MEDICAL MARIJUANA RECOMMENDATIONS FOR FIBROMYALGIA

Since fatigue is such a prominent symptom with FM, I recommend avoiding strong indica strains and high-CBD products, both of which might increase fatigue. The MMJ products and delivery methods that seem to work best for FM are:

- Topicals—generalized transdermal patches (1:1/CBD:THC—daytime; CBN—evening); and transdermal gel pens (CBD, THC, and CBN).
- Vaporizing hybrids—both 50:50 strains and sativa-dominant hybrids (60:40 and 70:30—if you can tolerate the psychoactive effect). I've also had some patients with FM who do well with a 60:40 indica-dominant strain.
- Edibles—hybrid and sativa.
- Topicals—localized (Apothecanna Extra Strength and Mary's Medicinals CBC seem to be most effective).
- Tinctures—1:1, 2:1, 3:1, or 6:1/CBD:THC.
- Tablets—both swallowed and sublingual; hybrids are best. Stratos tablets are available in both sativa (*Energy*) and hybrid (*Relax*), as well as 1:1 and 15:1/CBD:THC. Med-a-mints are also available in both sativa and hybrid sublingual tablets.

HOLISTIC MEDICAL TREATMENT AND PREVENTION PROGRAM FOR FIBROMYALGIA

Risk Factors and Causes

Although the cause of FM is unknown, most of the risk factors associated with chronic fatigue syndrome—especially food allergy (dairy products, wheat and gluten grains [barley, rye, and spelt], fermented foods, and nightshades [potatoes and eggplant] are most common), emotional stress, intestinal candida overgrowth, Lyme disease, nutritional deficiencies, and adrenal exhaustion—are also present with fibromyalgia. Research suggests that *damage to the cells' energy production in the mitochondria* (the energy production center of the cells), as a result of an excess of free radicals, is the primary cause of FM. Reduced circulation to muscle cells and low levels of the neurotransmitter serotonin may also contribute to FM. The metabolic shutdown in the muscle cells might possibly be due to the accumulation of phosphate and uric acid. Some of the standard medications (Zyloprim) used to treat gout (elevated uric acid) and other drugs that reduce uric acid and phosphate (Probenecid, Sulfinpyrazone, and Robinul) have significantly improved the well-being of some FM patients. It is now known that in people who have FM, the body breaks down muscle protein at an unusually high rate and converts it to glucose for energy. It has been theorized that this increased level of muscle tissue breakdown is one of the primary causes of the pain, aching, and fatigue. Aluminum and heavy metal toxicity may also play a role in causing FM.

The majority of fibromyalgia patients report that their symptoms came on following some type of trauma or severe infection. Many women with FM have a history of abuse. This can alter neurologic and hormonal response and create abnormal responses to stress—generally a heightened nervous system response that may create painful trigger points in the muscles.

Physical Health Recommendations for Fibromyalgia

Most people with fibromyalgia need some Functional Medicine testing to determine underlying imbalances.

The most important tests are for the following:

- Adrenal function.
- Stool and leaky gut.
- Food sensitivity.
- Nighttime neurotransmitters.
- Genetic detoxification and methylation, if you are chemically sensitive.

A holistic doctor can do these tests to determine the underlying causes of your syndrome.

The holistic treatment for FM is nearly identical to that of chronic fatigue syndrome.

Diet

The anti-inflammatory, candida-control diet described in Chapter 5 is recommended for FM. Avoiding gluten is *critical* if you have FM. Many patients feel significantly better after making just this one dietary change.

Vitamins, Minerals, and Supplements

- *Malic acid*: 1,200 to 2,400 mg daily, in combination with magnesium (300 to 600 mg daily), vitamin B6, and other synergistic factors. This product is available as Fibroplex from Metagenics. The recommended dosage is 2 tablets two to three times daily with food. These supplements help restore normal energy production in the muscle cells as well as aid in aluminum detoxification.
- *MitoVive* (Metagenics): Especially important to take for FM are vitamins and supplements that help to stimulate mitochondrial function. Recommended dosage is 1 scoop in water, one to two times daily between meals, especially before light exercise.
- *SeroSyn* (Metagenics): This product contains 5-HTP for increasing serotonin, which is deficient in most people with FM, along with skullcap, which helps ease pain, and ginseng for mental clarity. It can also help with sleep as well as overcome brain fog. Recommended dosage is 1 tablet three times daily at least ten to twenty minutes before meals.

- *NutraGems CoQ10* (Metagenics): 300 mg of super absorbable CoQ10 in a chewable gummy form. Recommended dosage is 1 serving daily at breakfast.
- *Intravenous vitamin and mineral injections*: These often produce significant improvement, and should be administered three or four times in a two-week period.
- *UltraClear RENEW* (Metagenics): Periodic seven- to twenty-one-day detox programs using this product have been shown in two clinical trials to greatly benefit FM patients as a result of its effect on leaky gut, enhancement of liver function, reduction of heavy metal toxicity, and reduction of free radical activity. Participants in studies had fewer tender points, more energy, less stiffness, and more flexibility. Ultra-Clear RENEW comes in the Clear Change detox kits that contain an instructional booklet and free online support.
- *PhytoMulti* (Metagenics): This product contains methylated B vitamins, antioxidants, minerals, and DNA-protecting plant extracts. Recommended dosage is 1 tablet two times daily with food.

Exercise

Exercise is an essential part of the treatment program for FM, but high-impact exercises such as jogging, basketball, or any other activity that involves jumping should be avoided. Ideal exercises include walking, a stationary bike or treadmill, swimming, qigong, t'ai chi, and yogic breathing. Another excellent type of exercise is the use of an AquaJogger. This is a buoyancy belt that fits around the chest and allows the person wearing it to stand up in a swimming pool and either walk or run against the resistance of the water.

Try to gradually work up to forty minutes of exercise, three times a week. You may have to begin with only five to ten minutes per exercise session. Learn to listen to your body, and do not push yourself to meet unrealistic goals. This is especially hard to do if you have been used to leading a very active, busy life. You must slow down and give your immune system a chance to heal.

Professional Care Therapies

Trigger point injections, IV nutrition (Myers' Cocktail), massage therapy, biofeedback, acupuncture, hydrotherapy, and electrostimulation have all been reported to be effective for some people with FM.

The Issues in Your Tissues

Almost all FM patients have a history of chronic *overdoing*. Not knowing their boundaries and limits is the hallmark of people suffering with FM. They often lack the ability to balance activity and rest.

If you are suffering from FM, you need to learn to say NO! You must create boundaries and strictly adhere to them. Stop trying to please and caretake others at your own expense. You cannot afford to ignore your needs and desires, and care for yourself as if you are "leftovers," as one patient described herself. You must make yourself the top priority in your life.

Counseling is strongly advised with FM patients. They need to learn to strike a healthier balance between work and relaxation along with establishing a slower pace, a healthier rhythm, in all of their activities. Learning to say no is vital to this process of healing.

FM support groups can be found locally through the *Fibromyalgia Network*, an organization based in Tucson, Arizona. Their phone number is (800-853-2929). The *Arthritis Foundation* in Atlanta, Georgia, also helps organize support groups and educational classes (844-571-HELP).

Patient Story—**Fibromyalgia and Migraine**

Leona H. is an unemployed twenty-nine-year-old diagnosed five years ago with fibromyalgia. She had been having symptoms for three years prior to her diagnosis. They began shortly after the unexpected death of her mother, leaving Leona as the oldest of three, to care for her teenage brothers. Her father was always busy working and spent very little time at home with his children.

Following her FM diagnosis, she was prescribed gabapentin, which was minimally effective for reducing her pain, but it made her too sleepy to function. Her primary symptoms are joint pain along with pain in her shoulders, neck, and upper back. Without MMJ, her pain level is a 7–8 and she's barely able to function. But after smoking or ingesting an indica, it is reduced to a 3–4. She often uses the topical cream Apothecanna Extra Strength, which has worked well for relieving the pain.

Leona has also had migraine headaches since the age of twelve. These too have responded well to MMJ. She had been having intense, incapacitating migraines approximately once a week, but now they've been reduced to one or two per month, with minimal pain, if she smokes a sativa within twenty to thirty minutes of the aura beginning.

She's currently seeing a therapist one to two times a month and is finding that to be quite helpful. The one time I saw Leona for the renewal of her MMJ license, in November 2016, she was shocked at how strongly she fit the personality profile of both the typical FM and the typical migraine patient. Her comment after hearing these descriptions of the "issues in the tissues" was "This is very helpful. It makes me feel like I have a lot more power to heal myself than I thought I had."

Chapter 10

GI Dis-ease: IBS, Crohn's Disease, and Ulcerative Colitis

Listen to Your Gut

The gastrointestinal tract provides the means by which we chew, digest, and obtain nourishment from food and eliminate indigestible fiber and wastes from the colon. Digestion starts in the mouth and continues in the stomach and small intestine. Most of the food's nutrients and water are absorbed through the intestinal wall while it is passing through the twenty-six-foot-long small bowel. In the large bowel (colon), remaining water and nutrients are absorbed into the bloodstream, leaving undigested food, toxins, and wastes for elimination. The normal transit time for food to travel from ingestion to stool passage is twelve to eighteen hours.

Over one thousand species of normal bacteria are found in the gastrointestinal tract, and the number of individual bacteria is more than ten times greater than the number of cells in the body (there are 37.2 trillion human body cells). Amazingly enough, the extensive system of lymph channels in the walls of the small bowel is the largest reservoir of immune function in the body. The intake of nutrients here profoundly influences the balance of the intestinal bacteria, potentially favoring growth of harmful microorganisms and profoundly affecting lymphatic and immune system function. This can then promote inflammation throughout the body.

The gastrointestinal tract also houses the body's "second brain," known as the enteric nervous system, located in the linings of the esophagus, stomach, small intestine, and colon. Scientists consider it a single entity—brimming with neurotransmitter proteins, produced by cells identical to those found in the brain. This complex circuitry enables the "G-I brain" (the "belly brain") to act independently, learn, remember, and *produce gut feelings*.

If the gut is imbalanced, it can profoundly affect your mood and energy. For example, the gut makes 90 percent of a neurotransmitter called serotonin—the "feel good" neurotransmitter. If the bacteria are imbalanced, then you are not able to properly manufacture serotonin, which could cause you to feel depressed, less resilient under stress, and more anxious, and cause you to have sleep problems.

Similarly, if you are feeling highly stressed for a prolonged period of time, it will have a significant impact on your belly brain and potentially create chronic digestive problems. This is especially true with irritable bowel syndrome, which not long ago was described by the medical community as a "temperamental bowel."

IRRITABLE BOWEL SYNDROME (IBS)

IBS, also called spastic or mucous colitis, is said to afflict over 20 percent of the American population. Women with IBS outnumber men two to one. IBS is the most frequent diagnosis made by gastroenterologists.

The symptoms are a result of hyper-function and malfunction of the gastrointestinal tract, involving the stomach, small intestine, and large bowel. The neural circuitry within the brain is probably involved as well.

The symptoms of irritable bowel syndrome include a change from normal bowel function to periods of diarrhea and constipation, often alternating, with belching, bloating, abdominal pain, nausea, loss of appetite, flatulence, and a feeling after a bowel movement that the bowel has not completely emptied.

IBS patients can either have constipation-dominant IBS (IBS-C) or diarrhea-dominant IBS (IBS-D). IBS-C is characterized by harder, dryer stools and skipping days of bowel movements, usually indicating a sluggish bowel. IBS-D produces diarrhea that is sometimes urgent, explosive, and nearly uncontrollable, may involve liquid stools with white mucous, and may occur immediately after a meal or soon after awakening in the morning, with large meals tending to aggravate symptoms.

Symptoms in women also tend to increase during premenstrual and menstrual phases of the cycle. Physical symptoms are often accompanied by notable depression and/or anxiety, and there is often the preexistence of psychological symptoms, which may worsen with the onset of the physical symptoms. Making the diagnosis requires exclusion of other causes of diarrhea and constipation.

MEDICAL MARIJUANA RECOMMENDATIONS FOR IBS, CROHN'S DISEASE, AND ULCERATIVE COLITIS

Anxiety is a major contributor to each of these GI conditions. As a result the focus of MMJ treatment is on reducing anxiety, in addition to relaxing the spasm in the smooth involuntary muscles controlling the peristaltic waves propelling food through the entire GI tract, and relieving the inflammation of the highly sensitive mucous membrane lining your gut.

Both *indica* and *high-CBD* products can address all three objectives quite well. Among my patients with these chronic GI problems, *edibles*, and especially *juicing* when possible (raw cannabis leaves are required) have been the preferred delivery methods. Direct contact with the mucosal lining seems to have a longer and stronger therapeutic effect than inhaling cannabis, although inhalation is also effective for relieving symptoms. Since cannabinoids can reduce motility of the bowel, some patients, especially those with IBS-C, find more effective relief when taking smaller "micro-doses" of the recommended products below.

For treating Crohn's and ulcerative colitis, I also recommend *THCa* (a powerful anti-inflammatory) in either a tincture or a transdermal patch. The following is a list of MMJ products and delivery methods helpful for all three GI conditions:

- Juicing raw cannabis leaves—for those without access to fresh plants, THCa tincture, CBDa tincture, and CBD tincture are excellent alternatives.

- Indica and hybrid edibles—gluten-free, without sugar or dairy
- Indica—especially edibles and vaporizing—60:40 or 70:30/I:S, during daytime hours, and stronger indicas (above 70:30) in the evening
- Vaporizing (daytime)—high-CBD strains of flower, especially Harlequin (a 50:50/I:S hybrid), Cannatonic (a 50:50 hybrid), or other hybrids (either 50:50 or 60:40/I:S)
- Topicals—generalized (apply to wrist or ankle for rapid absorption) transdermal patches, especially THCa, 3:2/CBDa:THCa, or 1:1/CBD:THC
- High-CBD tinctures—2:1, 3:1, or 6:1/CBD:THC
- Ingesting high-CBD hash oil—3:1, 6:1, 12:1, or higher/CBD:THC
- High-CBD sativa strains and THC may provide some relief to those GI patients also suffering with some degree of depression
- If depression is not a factor, then I would recommend avoiding sativa and high-THC products

HOLISTIC MEDICAL TREATMENT AND PREVENTION PROGRAM FOR IBS

Risk Factors and Causes

Most gastroenterologists believe the cause of irritable bowel syndrome is unknown. The following factors are thought by many holistic physicians to be contributory:

- Food sensitivity or allergy—most often, in order of frequency, milk and milk derivatives, wheat and gluten grains (barley, rye, oats, and spelt), coffee, chocolate, citrus fruits, corn, eggs, nuts, and potatoes
- Intolerance of sugars—fructose, sucrose, sorbitol, mannitol, and lactose (in milk).
- SIBO—Recently there have been several studies showing that some people who have been diagnosed with IBS may actually have a condition called SIBO: small intestinal bacterial overgrowth—*especially if bloating is the dominant symptom.* This is caused by an overgrowth of two of the predominant types of bacteria in the small intestine. They ferment certain carbohydrates in food, producing excess hydrogen or methane gas, which causes bloating.

- Bacterial infections—might be low-grade and require highly sensitive stool testing.
- Parasitic intestinal infestation—incidence estimate by some authorities as high as 30–50 percent in IBS.
- Candida (yeast) overgrowth—treatment with antifungal drugs and/ or supplements shown to result in great improvement in IBS patients not responsive to food elimination diets.
- Pancreatic enzyme insufficiency—pancreatic enzymes are not secreted in sufficient amounts in response to food, creating more chance for food to ferment or putrefy, therefore affecting gas, bloating, and the motility of the intestine, which can then slow down the movement of food through the intestine.
- Psychological and social stress—creating accelerated motility of the colon in IBS patients experiencing it.

For more in-depth information on the causes of IBS, gas, and bloating, download the free report titled *The 7 Causes of Gas and Bloating and What You Can Do About It*, by Todd Nelson, naturopath, at www .tolwellness.com.

Physical Health Recommendations

Successful treatment begins with a thorough *investigation for possible causes and triggers* of IBS:

- Careful search for bacterial and parasitic organisms, and a digestive stool analysis utilizing a Functional Medicine laboratory especially equipped for sensitive and comprehensive testing of stool specimens; specific treatment then follows for any abnormal organisms found on testing.
- Tracking of triggering foods and emotional stress factors you suspect might impact the waxing and waning pattern of IBS symptoms, done by diet/symptom journal-keeping, which includes recording foods you've eaten, bowel movement timing, consistency of stools, and how your gut feels, from which you will quickly learn what foods to avoid and what to include.
- Intestinal permeability functional testing for leaky gut syndrome. (There are several labs that do blood testing for this. See Resources.)

- Hydrogen/methane breath challenge test for small intestine bacterial overgrowth to determine if you have SIBO.
- Food sensitivity testing—blood testing from a highly specialized Functional Medicine lab (see Resources).

Diet

Besides the dietary guidelines in Chapter 5, dietary considerations in IBS include the following:

- For IBS-D, begin with the gradual addition of *high fiber* from primarily steamed vegetables and vegetable soups. Only add raw vegetables and fruit if you are sure they won't loosen stools or increase bowel movement frequency. Only include beans and lentils if tolerated, adding one to two new foods per week, making careful observation of the tolerance of each.
- Unprocessed *psyllium seed powder* gradually increased from one rounded teaspoonful to two tablespoons daily tends to stabilize the loose bowel habit. Don't use wheat or other cereal bran, as it may aggravate the problem if sensitivity to these grains is present. Brown rice may be the best grain, as it may slow down BMs and help form the stool.
- The intake of *water* should be six to eight glasses daily, sufficient to keep the urine very pale yellow most of the time.
- Thorough *chewing* and unhurried eating in a relaxed atmosphere are encouraged.
- Sugar is discouraged. Studies have shown that intestinal motility is prolonged by nearly *two and one-half times over normal* after introduction of a high load of sugar. This disruption of intestinal motility is one of the main problems in IBS. Sugar also encourages growth of candida (yeast), which has been implicated as an additional contributing factor in IBS.

Supplements—IBS-D

- *ProbioMax Plus DF* (Xymogen): This powerful probiotic in individual premeasured servings contains different strains of highly researched acidophilus and bifidus, along with *Saccharomyces boulardii* and immunoglobulin proteins derived from colostrum. It is exceptional in helping reduce diarrhea and loose stools. Empty one packet in water and drink before bed. It may also be taken first thing in the morning. Once bowels are more stable, then switch to *ProbioMax Daily* (Xymogen): 1 capsule on an empty stomach before bed. If needed, you can also take 1 capsule in the morning.

- *Glutagenics* (Metagenics): This is a powdered combination of L-glutamine, DGL licorice, and freeze-dried aloe vera. The combination of these three ingredients helps soothe and repair the gut lining, and heal a leaky gut. Take 1 rounded teaspoon in water, morning and night, on an empty stomach, for two to six months.
- Other supplements need to be personalized depending on the Functional Medicine lab test results. For example, you may need herbs to kill infections, or pancreatic enzymes if you are found to be deficient in those.

Supplements—IBS-C

- *UltraFlora IB* (Metagenics): 60 billion beneficial bacteria per capsule and highly effective for those suffering from constipation with IBS. Start with 1 capsule morning and night, on an empty stomach, for three weeks, then try reducing to 1 capsule before bed.
- *Mag Citrate* (Metagenics): The muscular action of the intestine (peristalsis) is dependent on magnesium, which acts as a gentle laxative. Start with 200–300 mg before dinner or at bedtime. You can gradually increase the dose until you experience a loose stool, then slowly reduce the dose until you are having more regular stools.
- *Glutagenics* (Metagenics): as described in the supplements for IBS-D.

Supplements—IBS-D and IBS-C

- *UltraGI Replenish* (Metagenics): a medical food. The recommended dosage is two scoops one to two times daily; contraindicated if SIBO is present.

Food Sensitivity

A food elimination and re-challenge trial should be undertaken if food sensitivity suspicion is high. You can also avoid extended food trials and simply try omitting the more highly suspect foods listed under "Risk Factors and Causes" earlier. Other less common offenders include tea and onions. Placed on a low-antigenic diet limited to a few foods, IBS patients commonly feel much improved within a week. Since food additives can occasionally be a problem, organically grown foods are desirable. *Of those who follow a carefully planned exclusion diet, 75 percent experience substantial improvement.*

If SIBO is diagnosed, you need to strictly avoid eating certain fermentable carbohydrates that will contribute to bloating, gas, and discomfort. You want to starve the offending bacteria, kill them with a strong professional herbal compound, and restore the bacterial balance. This should all be done under the supervision of a holistic doctor. A good educational website about SIBO is www.siboinfo.com.

Herbs

Intesol (Metagenics)—enteric-coated capsules containing peppermint oil, chamomile extract, and lavender oil. A German study found clinical improvement and decrease in pain to be twice as great from peppermint oil compared to a placebo. This combination is antispasmodic and can help reduce gas. Take 1 capsule before each meal. Do NOT take if you have esophageal reflux (GERD)/heartburn, since peppermint oil can make it worse.

A mixture of twenty Chinese herbs, including *Artemesiae capillaris*, *Codonopsis pilosula*, *Coicis lachyrma-jobi*, *Atractylodis macrocephalae*, *Schisandra*, and others, was recently shown to be of substantial help with IBS symptoms. Herbal teas with antispasmodic properties (chamomile, peppermint, rosemary, and valerian) are soothing. Robert's Formula is also helpful in treatment (see under "Crohn's Disease" below).

The Issues in Your Tissues

IBS has been linked to the mental and emotional issues of gut-level fear, distrust, low self-confidence, personal honor, and self-care. There is a tendency for IBS patients to be highly invested in control and self-criticism, and an effort needs to be made to modify the attitudes behind these thoughts and behaviors. Dealing with and resolving the issues surrounding the early childhood origin of these traits is most beneficial. Working to improve the quality of sleep also reaps significant benefits in bringing symptoms under control. Irritable bowel syndrome patients are often worriers, with special concern about work and their disease. Fun, play, and laughter can be highly therapeutic.

Stressful incidents and increased levels of self-imposed pressure are frequently associated with flare-ups of IBS. These recurrences can be modified by insight-oriented psychotherapy, particularly successful when augmented by *relaxation training* and practice with *biofeedback*. Some studies have documented 75 percent improvement in physical and psychological symptoms after several months of regular biofeedback practice. *Hypnosis* is also very effective with irritable bowel syndrome. After an initial series of treatments, the best results occur in patients who periodically—one to three times a year—return for a session of re-inforcement. *Self-affirmations* are particularly effective, especially when repeated during relaxation, biofeedback, or *meditation*. An example: *My intestine is healed and is serving me well.*

Patient Story—IBS

John K. is a twenty-eight-year-old tech system administrator whose symptoms began at the age of twenty-one, shortly after he began commuting almost two hours round-trip to attend college. He describes this as a very stressful time in his life, both the pressure of the academics and the long commute. Driving long distances significantly increased his anxiety level, which was high to begin with. Associated with the commute, he was making more frequent stops at fast-food restaurants.

His early symptoms were moderate to severe abdominal pain, quickly followed by diarrhea. His visits to physicians were focused on ruling out more serious GI problems, before he was finally given the diagnosis of IBS. The medications he was given were largely ineffective, and he found his greatest relief with smoking marijuana.

This was 2009, the same year Colorado made medical marijuana legally available for sale. Having already experienced the medical benefit of marijuana in a state where it was illegal, he decided to move from Pennsylvania to Colorado.

He began using MMJ shortly after arriving in Boulder, and although it was quite effective for relieving his symptoms once they began, he was still having pain with diarrhea almost daily. Moving from home, he found himself feeling lonely and anxious, in a place where he knew no one. He also started a new job.

It took several years for him to recognize the triggers for his discomfort. When I saw him recently for the renewal of his MMJ license, he felt better and more in control of his GI dis-ease than at any time since it began seven years ago. He had identified several foods, especially red meat and greasy foods, that triggered his symptoms.

When I saw him a year ago, he was quite pleased with his improvement, primarily due to vaporizing or smoking indica strains after work. They helped him to relax and to reduce anxiety and the frequency and intensity of his pain. On his latest visit he reported even greater improvement than the year before. He had found a new MMJ product, the Stratos tablet (1:1/CBD:THC). This product is comparable to an edible in duration (six to eight hours), and John felt that the tablets were more effective than the strains of indica flower he'd been smoking previously.

Earlier this year, he also began seeing a psychotherapist on a weekly basis to help relieve his anxiety. The counseling, together with the MMJ tablets, modifying his diet to eliminate the trigger foods, and sleeping better, has made a huge difference in the quality of John's life. He also feels as if he has a much greater sense of control, and he's clearly a happier guy than when I first met him.

CROHN'S DISEASE

Crohn's disease is a bowel disorder involving inflammation of the entire wall of the small and large intestine, but most impacted is the terminal ileum (the last one-third of the small bowel) as it empties into the colon.

Both Crohn's disease and ulcerative colitis are considered *inflammatory bowel disease* (IBD). Crohn's disease is an autoimmune condition, estimated to afflict more than one hundred thousand people in the United States. A slight majority are women. Age of onset is usually between fifteen and forty. Inflammatory bowel disease is more than twice as common in Caucasians than in non-Caucasians and four times as common in Jews than in non-Jews, and since the 1950s there has been a steady, remarkable increase in the incidence of Crohn's disease in the United States.

The predominant symptom of Crohn's is pain in the lower abdomen (usually the right side), often accompanied by episodes of diarrhea, mild fever, loss of appetite, weight loss, flatulence, and a general feeling of malaise or being unwell.

Crohn's disease leads to a distorted pattern of assimilation of nutrients from the affected segments of the small bowel. The levels of pro-inflammatory prostaglandins, including the extremely potent leukotrienes, are greatly elevated in the wall of the affected bowel. Abnormal bacteria and yeast organisms often overgrow the small intestine, creating secondary problems. Protein is not properly absorbed, and this leads to weight loss in many cases. The complications of Crohn's—liver, skin, spine, and joint problems, probably stem from the abnormal assimilation of proteins due to the disease itself. As a result of losses from diarrhea or poor assimilation through the inflamed mucosal lining, it is common in Crohn's disease to have *low levels* of:

- Vitamins A, C, D, E, and K
- B-complex vitamins—B12 deficient 50 percent of the time; folic acid deficient 25–65 percent of the time
- Magnesium, potassium, calcium
- Iron—dropped levels due to bleeding from inflamed mucosal lesions
- Trace minerals—zinc deficient in 40 percent of Crohn's patients

HOLISTIC MEDICAL TREATMENT AND PREVENTION PROGRAM FOR CROHN'S DISEASE

Risk Factors and Causes

- Genetic predisposition (20–40 percent of patients)
- Immunological abnormalities
- Emotional stress
- Infection
- Dietary factors

- Ingestion of excess food allergens, hybridized wheat, and GMO foods sprayed with glyphosate (Roundup), a popular pesticide

The presence of antibodies to a bacterium, *Klebsiella*, is found in a high percentage of Crohn's patients and patients who have rheumatoid spondylitis of the spine (a spinal arthritis). In fact, men with Crohn's are more prone to develop spondylitis. Some physicians believe these facts favor an infectious cause of both diseases. Crohn's is also associated with arthritis of other joints—wrists, knees, and ankles. Inflammatory skin nodules and canker sores are also more common in Crohn's patients.

Crohn's disease and ulcerative colitis are extremely rare in primitive societies not consuming calorie-dense, highly refined, Westernized diets. This dietary influence is significant. The diets of people who subsequently develop Crohn's disease have been documented to contain substantially less fruit, vegetables, and fiber and to include far more sugar and refined flour foods compared to those who remain healthy. One study found that the amount of sugar consumed by those who later got Crohn's disease was twice that of healthy matched controls.

Physical Health Recommendations

Diet

Review the anti-inflammatory diet in Chapter 5.

Since the predisposing low-fiber, highly refined carbohydrate intake is considered a significant risk factor for developing Crohn's, the diet of choice removes sugar and refined flour, gluten (especially hybridized wheat), and GMO foods such as corn and soy, and adds fiber from vegetables, fruits, and gluten-free whole grains such as rice, quinoa, millet, and buckwheat. If you are having frequent loose stools, most vegetables should be steamed or in soups. If you cannot tolerate raw fruits, then try applesauce, bananas, and pears. You should greatly reduce or eliminate meat and dairy products to diminish levels of leukotrienes and inflammation, especially if the meat is commercially raised with antibiotics and other additives. Eat only chemical-free, organic meats. If you continue to eat beef, make sure it's from grass-fed cows, not cows that are ingesting

GMO corn. Increase intake of ocean fish (for example, salmon, sole, cod, halibut, and mackerel), with two to four servings each week.

Vitamins, Minerals, and Supplements

- *UltraInflamX Plus 360* (Metagenics): I strongly recommend drinking this medical food powder. It has been highly effective in patients with inflammatory bowel disease. This should only be done under the supervision of a holistic practitioner.
- *Multivitamin/mineral/antioxidant/phytonutrient formula*: Take an easy-to-absorb one, such as PhytoMulti from Metagenics: 1 tablet with meals, two times daily.
- *Vitamin A*: Take 50,000 IU daily during the acute phase or reactivation of the disease. This should be monitored by a practitioner.
- *Vitamin C*: Take 1–2 gm daily; magnesium, potassium, and calcium ascorbate in Ester-C forms are often less irritating to the bowel.
- *Vitamin D3*: Make sure your blood level of vitamin D is optimized at 70–80 ng/ml. Until you have a blood test, you can take a maintenance dose of 5,000 IU of D3 daily with food.
- *E Complex-1:1* (Metagenics): Take 2 softgels with one meal daily.
- *Quercetin*: Take 0.5–1 gm three to four times daily.
- *Methyl Protect* (Xymogen): This provides exceptional methylated forms of folate and B12 that are easily absorbed. Take 1 tablet two to three times daily with food.
- *Zinc A. G.* (Metagenics): Take 1 pill twice daily with a meal.
- *Mag Glycinate* (Metagenics): This is a well-tolerated bowel product. Take 1 tablet at breakfast and 2 with dinner.
- *Glutagenics* (Metagenics): For restoring gut lining health, take 1 rounded teaspoon two to three times daily in water between meals.
- *Fish oil* (OmegaGenics EPA-DHA 2400 from Metagenics): This reduces the frequency of relapses by 40–50 percent. OmegaGenics is a very strong, economical, pleasant-tasting liquid fish oil. Take 1 teaspoon two times daily with a meal.
- *OmegaGenics SPM Active* (Metagenics): A fish-oil derivative that accelerates the resolution of inflammation. Begin with a loading dose of 2 capsules three times a day with food for one to two weeks. Then

reduce to 2 capsules twice a day for three weeks, followed by a maintenance dose of 1–4 capsules a day.

- *Flaxseed oil*: Contains ALA omega 3 oil. Take one tablespoonful daily.
- *Adequate protein*: This is conveniently supplied in *amino acid* supplements that are derived from foods unlikely to be offending (milk and wheat) and require no digestion before assimilation. Pea and rice protein concentrate will meet this need with a very low chance of allergic reaction (UltraGI Replenish from Metagenics).
- *Gamma oryzanol*: Take 100 mg three to four times daily (derived from rice bran oil). This is readily available in health food stores.

Herbs

Commonly used herbs include *marshmallow root*, *wild indigo*, *ginger*, *goldenseal*, and *slippery elm*. These are often combined in a traditional naturopathic formulation, Robert's Formula, that you can get from a naturopath or holistic doctor. It is advisable to consult a health professional for a balanced program before using these botanicals.

The Issues in Your Tissues

Stress plays a major role with Crohn's disease, just as it does with nearly every one of the most common chronic pain conditions. The issues in the tissues contributing heavily to Crohn's are very similar to those associated with IBS (see above). All inflammatory conditions and immune responses improve with the reduction of stress that follows consistent practice of *relaxation skills*, *biofeedback*, and *meditation*. It cannot be overemphasized: the mind is infinitely more powerful than we can imagine.

Patient Stories—**Crohn's Disease**

Coltyn T. is a very mature and articulate sixteen-year-old high school sophomore who has had Crohn's disease since the age of nine. By eleven, he was incapacitated and in a wheelchair. Surgery to remove most of his ileum was recommended, but he declined. As a result of a highly aggressive pharmaceutical treatment regimen, including high-dose steroids and extremely painful injections of Humira, he developed rheumatoid arthritis and lupus.

At his suggestion, his family moved from Illinois to Colorado in order to gain access to medical marijuana (prior to its legalization in Illinois). After seven months on cannabis, taking capsules of hash oil (containing 15 mg THC plus 15 mg CBD) four times a day, Coltyn was in complete remission. He has remained on that regimen for the past two years and "feels great," with almost no symptoms of Crohn's, RA, or lupus. He has also become a passionate proponent for MMJ.

Alyssa C. is a twenty-six-year-old mental health worker who had been in excellent health until one and a half years before when she was initially diagnosed with Crohn's disease. Only a few months later she developed rheumatoid arthritis, and began treatment with Humira, two (very painful) injections every two weeks; plus prednisone (a corticosteroid) at a dosage of 60 mg daily, which she was to gradually taper over twelve months. Within several weeks of beginning this treatment regimen, she developed adrenal failure from the prednisone, and decided to stop both medications. She currently takes no prescription drugs.

Her MMJ daily regimen consists of the following:

- CBD capsules—25 mg two times a day
- Stratos Relax (hybrid) tablets—one or two times a day
- THCa tincture—once daily
- Vaporizing—either a hybrid or an indica in the evening

She has modified her diet to strict vegetarian and gluten-free, with no oils except olive and coconut. She takes the following supplements on a daily basis: vitamins A, C, and D; calcium, magnesium glycinate, activated charcoal, amino acids, ginger, and turmeric; an essential oil blend consisting of peppermint, tarragon, and ginger; and Glutagenics (Metagenics).

She has been essentially symptom-free (from Crohn's and RA) for much of the past year on her current MMJ/holistic regimen. The day before seeing me for the renewal of her MMJ license, she had a colonoscopy performed by her gastroenterologist (the first one had been done at the time her diagnosis was made, a year and a half earlier). The result: "He was blown away by what he saw. There was *no inflammation*!"

ULCERATIVE COLITIS

Ulcerative colitis is a chronic inflammatory disease of the large bowel (colon), occasionally affecting the lower part of the small bowel. The inflammation of the bowel wall is so intense that ulcer-like erosions of the tissue lining the bowel are created.

Upward of four hundred thousand people in the United States are thought to have ulcerative colitis. Onset is typically between the ages of fifteen and thirty-five. It strikes women more often than men, Caucasians more often than blacks, and those of Jewish descent more often than others. Like Crohn's, it is rarely seen in indigenous peoples.

The most frequent symptoms of ulcerative colitis are bloody diarrhea, low abdominal cramps, loss of appetite, and sometimes fever. Malaise and weight loss are common. The highly inflamed and ulcerated surface bleeds extremely easily. A common pattern ensues in which phases of partial healing are interrupted by acute relapses.

Conventional medical treatment of both ulcerative colitis and Crohn's disease typically includes a sulfa antibiotic, Azulfidine (sulfasalazine), and often large doses of corticosteroids (prednisone) to suppress the inflammation in more severe cases. The dosages of prednisone or other potent synthetic cortisone derivatives are then slowly tapered off to avoid the long-term serious consequences of steroids in the body. These side effects include:

- Suppression of the immune system
- Overgrowth of yeast organisms in the intestine
- Osteoporosis
- Weight gain that spares the limbs
- Moon-faced appearance
- Development of prominent blood vessels in the skin
- Wasting of muscle protein
- Promotion of diabetes
- Loss of neuronal connections in areas of the brain

Rarely, all medical measures fail, and surgical removal of the colon or diseased portions of it becomes a necessary life-saving measure. Patients who have relapsing ulcerative colitis for fifteen to twenty years are at a higher risk for the development of cancer of the bowel and rectum and need regular assessment because of this.

HOLISTIC MEDICAL TREATMENT AND PREVENTION PROGRAM FOR ULCERATIVE COLITIS

Risk Factors and Causes

The cause of ulcerative colitis is currently unknown; the following are possible contributors:

- Genetic factors
- Infectious agents—numerous theories implicate viruses or bacteria as a cause.
- Nutritional factors—inflammatory bowel diseases are seen scarcely, if at all, in indigenous cultures on whole food diets.
- Food allergies and food sensitivity—although this is not usually mentioned in conventional textbooks, the consistent substantial improvement with treatment by elimination and exclusion diets, or parenteral feedings (intravenous nutrition only, with nothing by mouth), lends strong support to this possibility.
- Disorders of the gut microbiome and imbalances in bowel bacteria may be a contributor.
- Immunity—the immune theory classifies ulcerative colitis as an autoimmune disease similar to rheumatoid arthritis and lupus erythematosus. Anti-colon antibodies have been demonstrated in some studies, lending support to this view.
- Psychological and emotional factors appear to play a significant contributory role in this disease.

Carrageenan, a commonly used food stabilizer in the nutrition industry, induces ulcerative colitis in guinea pigs. It may exert its damage when combined with the presence of a specific bacterium, *Bacteroides vulgatus.* The latter is six times more common in ulcerative colitis patients compared to normal healthy controls. *Carrageenan should be avoided in ulcerative colitis patients until further research information on this question emerges.*

Comprehensive testing is recommended for the functional status of the intestine and bowel. If pathogenic organisms (bacteria or parasites) are identified, specific treatment is as follows.

Physical Health Recommendations

Bowel rest is recommended in the acute phase of the disease. With severe symptoms, nutrition needs to be supplied by products that yield low fiber residual, reducing the stimulation and work required by the diseased bowel, such as UltraGI Replenish by Metagenics, or MediPro by Thorne Research (Dover, Idaho). In more severe cases of acute onset, intravenous feedings with nothing by mouth for a few days is necessary to sufficiently rest the bowel.

Diet

Caloric malnutrition often occurs because of poor assimilation of nutrients and declining appetite. This is more common when diarrhea is severe; optimum treatment makes use of a higher fiber diet without utilizing wheat bran.

A *food elimination* protocol is recommended to confirm or rule out food sensitivity as a possible cause of ulcerative colitis. When food sensitivity is found to be the central issue, as it is in some colitis patients, appropriate exclusions from the diet bring great and long-lasting improvement. Occasionally, the elimination of offending foods is *permanently curative.* In general, elimination of dairy products, sugar, and wheat is a likely place to start. Other more commonly found offenders are eggs, corn, cocoa, peanuts, oranges, soy, pork, beef, and chicken. Coffee, although it is a non-food, belongs on the list as well. Following a food elimination program is time and effort well spent.

Vitamins, Minerals, and Supplements

High amounts of micronutrient support are necessary in the acute and chronic phases of this disease. A potent, daily, megadose multivitamin-mineral combination needs to include high amounts of antioxidant *vitamins C, D, E, K,* and *B12* and *folic acid.* I recommend PhytoMulti from Metagenics and a dosage of 1 tablet twice daily with food. Azulfidine, if used long-term, hastens the loss of folic acid, and extra intake is necessary. *PABA* (para-aminobenzoic acid), a B-complex vitamin manifesting anti-inflammatory and anti-fibrotic effects, is effective in doses of 2 gm four times daily.

Mineral deficiencies are common in inflammatory bowel disease of all kinds; anemia and iron deficiency are common because of persistent bleeding; extra losses of calcium, magnesium, potassium, and zinc occur with diarrhea. The PhytoMulti mentioned above should provide basic, broad-spectrum nutrients that are easily absorbed. In addition, you might want to consider adding:

- *Vitamin B12*: Take 1,000 mcg of methylcobalamin in a sublingual lozenge.
- *Vitamin C or magnesium-potassium-calcium ascorbate*: Take 1–2 gm daily.
- *Vitamin D3*: Take 5,000 IU daily. (Have your vitamin D level checked periodically with a blood test.)
- *Vitamin E*: Take 800 IU daily.
- *OmegaGenics SPM Active* (Metagenics): Same dosage recommendations as for Crohn's.
- *Folate*: 3–5 mg daily. (I recommend 5-MTHF [Xymogen] 1,000 mcg one to five times per day.)
- *Quercetin*: $\frac{1}{2}$–1 gm three to four times daily.
- *Glutagenics* (Metagenics): 1 teaspoon three times daily for two months, then reduced to twice daily for another three months. (This will help to heal the gut lining.)
- *Hemagenics* (Metagenics): 1 tablet two to three times daily with food if iron is low and you are anemic.
- *OSAplex* (Xymogen): Take 1 packet two times daily with food for easily digested forms of calcium, magnesium, vitamin D3, and vitamin K for bone health.
- *Zinc A. G.* (Metagenics): 50 mg twice daily with food.
- *Potassium*: 500–700 mg daily.

- *Gamma oryzanol*: 100 mg three times daily for four to six weeks.
- *Dehydroepiandrosterone* (DHEA): If levels are low, modest replacement doses are helpful, usually 10–20 mg daily for women and 15–25 mg daily for men.

Herbs

Herbal remedies not yet subjected to controlled studies but long in common use to treat ulcerative colitis include *goldenseal* (2–3 capsules four times a day in the acute phase) and Robert's Formula, or its modification Bastyr Formula, from Eclectic Institute or NF Formulas.

In healthy people, the mucous blanket that protects the intestinal surface contains mucins that have been found to be distinctly abnormal in active phases of ulcerative colitis yet normal in remission. Herbs that are helpful in promoting mucus secretion are *deglycyrrhizinated licorice-DGL* (found in Glutagenics, mentioned above), *slippery elm*, and *marshmallow root*.

The Issues in Your Tissues

Stress. Physicians familiar with many cases of ulcerative colitis see a consistent pattern, with onset often associated with some acutely stressful life event. Large studies have linked recurrences to the stopping of smoking. Why would smoking deter the recurrence of this illness? If the stress theory is accepted, one can theorize that smoking might be an outlet for the expression of tension and anxiety; when that outlet is no longer available, the stress-generated responses find their way to expression in the body.

The answer lies in the incorporation of the excellent techniques that are helpful in nearly all disease: the relaxed state achieved through the practice of biofeedback, meditation, imagery, quiet contemplation, autogenics, or progressive relaxation. Hypnotherapy too, particularly in conjunction with other methods, can be of enormous assistance.

Extensive early studies of ulcerative colitis patients showed that the conversations of subjects, especially at times of recurrences, were often sprinkled with statements expressing a desire to get rid of their stressful troubles. Ulcerative colitis and diarrhea have been found in numerous studies and clinical experience to be related to high levels of anger, particularly when the patient possesses no socially acceptable skill for the expression of his or her hostility. If you have ulcerative colitis, even the chance to talk about your feelings, without acting them out, may be a novel experience for you.

The *attitude* most often underlying the emotional experience of anger is hostility; indeed, ulcerative colitis patients are found to have tendencies toward hostility, conformity, and rigidity more often than comparison subjects without ulcerative colitis. Ulcerative colitis is also one of the diseases in which the initial episode is often associated with the loss of an important relationship. Appropriate counseling and personal work to help alter the psychological dynamics, attitudes, and worldview under which you are functioning can have an enormous payoff, with lessening of symptoms and normalization of bowel function. Clearly, ulcerative colitis is one of the many gastrointestinal dysfunctions that are more than organ-specific problems. These dysfunctions are only local manifestations of a systemic or generalized problem, which has many aspects—mental, emotional, nutritional, hereditary, allergic, neurological, and hormonal. To approach anything resembling a cure frequently requires a comprehensive, holistic approach.

Patient Story—**Ulcerative Colitis**

Michele B. is a sixty-two-year-old self-employed small-business owner (computer repair/website building), with a sixteen-year history of ulcerative colitis. After being diagnosed in 2001 (at the time, she had just completed several courses of antibiotics for a dental infection, and was also experiencing lots of stress), she was prescribed Asacol and prednisone. The prednisone "made me crazy, with bizarre behavior and major mood swings. I had to stop taking it." The other recommended medications were Humira and methotrexate, which she said were "horrible."

Following the diagnosis, she stopped smoking cigarettes and began investigating more natural treatments, such as diet and supplements. However, she continued having colitis attacks, with severe diarrhea, bleeding, gas, and bloating that could last for months. Since MMJ became available in Colorado in 2009, she's been using it daily and her attacks have gradually become much less severe (no bleeding or pain) and less frequent, occurring approximately two to three times a year. And they last no longer than one to two weeks.

She currently ingests hybrid or indica edibles on a daily basis, and occasionally smokes or vaporizes hybrids for pain. In July 2016 she experienced a shamanic long-distance energy healing, and was in complete remission for over four months before having a mild attack triggered by stress. She's aware that her diet has a significant impact on the severity of the attacks but "it's definitely stress that triggers them."

Chapter 11

Musculoskeletal (M-S) Pain: Knees, Neck, Shoulders, and Hips
What's the Message?

Pain that affects the bones, joints, cartilage, muscles, and tendons is considered musculoskeletal pain. Osteoarthritis and low back pain (Chapters 6 and 7) are the most frequent types of M-S pain for which patients seek medical treatment. The bulk of the common musculoskeletal pain conditions affect the knees, neck, shoulders (especially rotator cuff injury), hips, spine, wrists (especially carpal tunnel syndrome), and ankles, and are diagnosed as sprains, strains, tears, fractures, and tendinitis.

Sports- and work-related injuries, motor vehicle accidents, orthopedic surgery, or overuse of the affected joint or body part are the most common causes of M-S pain cited among the patients seeking treatment with medical marijuana. Athough the human body is a self-healing organism, for a variety of reasons this painful condition is *not* healing in these particular patients. Of all chronic pain conditions, musculoskeletal pain is among the most challenging to treat, for both conventional and holistic medicine.

Opioids and NSAIDs, both prescription (Naproxen, Celebrex) and over-the-counter (ibuprofen), are the drugs of choice for physicians treating patients suffering with chronic M-S pain.

MEDICAL MARIJUANA RECOMMENDATIONS
FOR MUSCULOSKELETAL PAIN

The MMJ recommendations are essentially the same as those for osteo-arthritis, with the exception of a greater emphasis on treating inflam-mation in those suffering with arthritis. Nearly all forms of M-S pain have an inflammatory component, but it is not typically as severe as it is with arthritis.

- Topicals—localized (apply to painful joints), especially Apothecanna Extra Strength or Mary's Medicinals CBC.
- Topicals—generalized (apply to wrist or ankle for rapid absorption) transdermal patches, especially 1:1/CBD:THC, 3:2/CBDa:THCa, and THCa; also Mary's Medicinals transdermal gel pens, CBD, THC, or CBN.
- Vaporizing high-CBD strains of flower—especially Harlequin (a 50:50/S:I hybrid), Lucy (a 70:30/I:S indica), Cannatonic (a 50:50 hybrid), or other hybrids (either 50:50, 60:40/S:I, or 60:40/I:S).
- High-CBD tinctures—1:1, 2:1, or 3:1/CBD:THC.
- High-CBD hash oil—3:1 or 6:1/CBD:THC.
- Juicing raw cannabis leaves—for those without access to fresh plants, THCa tincture, CBDa tincture, and CBD tincture are excellent alter-natives.
- Indica strains of flower—I:S of 70:30 or above (also good for sleep).
- Indica and hybrid edibles—gluten-free, without sugar or dairy (indica edibles are also good for sleep).
- Any strain or MMJ product containing CBG.

NOTE: Avoid sativa strains above 60:40/S:I and high-THC products. Although THC has both analgesic and anti-inflammatory properties, it can also increase anxiety, which has the potential to increase pain. If spasticity is a prominent symptom, then THC may be beneficial.

HOLISTIC MEDICAL TREATMENT AND PREVENTION PROGRAM FOR MUSCULOSKELETAL PAIN

Physical Health Recommendations

Diet

Diet can play a significant role in reducing M-S pain due to the fact that inflammation is an important contributor. The anti-inflammatory and alkalinizing diet presented in Chapter 5 is recommended. I suggest you pay particular attention to the "Acid/Alkaline Food Chart" and reduce highly acidic foods from your diet.

Vitamins, Minerals, and Supplements

If your M-S pain involves a joint or cartilage, then I would suggest you adhere to the recommendations and dosages in Chapter 6 for osteo-arthritis, including:

- *Wellness Essentials Active Packets* (Metagenics): These contain *glucosamine sulfate* and *chondroitin sulfate*, both of which help to build new cartilage.
- *Essential fatty acids, flaxseed oil, and MSM*: All of which will reduce inflammation.
- *Vitamin D3*: See the recommendations for vitamin D in Chapter 5.

Exercise

Yoga can be especially beneficial as part of the treatment program for M-S pain. The exercise you choose should avoid repeated impact of an affected joint—e.g., no running or jumping if you're healing a painful knee, hip, or ankle. If it's your shoulder, neck, back, or wrists, I would recommend you avoid weight training. Brisk walking, as long as it does not exacerbate the pain, is a good option, along with swimming.

Professional Care Therapies

Conventional medicine relies heavily on physical therapy to treat patients suffering with chronic musculoskeletal pain, and for many patients this can be quite helpful. However, as I explained in Chapter 7 with respect to chronic low back pain and yoga, it is usually most effective if the patient continues doing the physical therapy exercises and stretches at home on a daily basis.

In addition there are many complementary therapies that are helpful for relieving chronic M-S pain, including: traditional Chinese medicine, especially acupuncture and Chinese herbs; Ayurvedic medicine, especially Boswellin Cream, camphor, and eucalyptus oil; bodywork (Rolfing, Hellerwork, and the Loren Berry Method); body movement therapies (Feldenkrais and Pilates); chiropractic and osteopathic manipulation (can increase circulation to a painful joint); homeopathy; and craniosacral therapy.

Energy medicine therapies such as *Healing Touch* or *Reiki* are among the most beneficial for treating M-S pain. Energy medicine is a comprehensive approach to healing that features all interactions between body, mind, and environment, including magnetic, electric, electromagnetic, acoustic, chemical, physical, and gravitational factors.

Healing Touch is a holistic energy medicine therapy utilizing a variety of hands-on techniques to balance and realign the energy within and surrounding the body. As a Healing Touch practitioner, some of my most successful and dramatic treatment outcomes have occurred with patients suffering from long-term musculoskeletal pain—knees, shoulders, back, and wrists.

The Issues in Your Tissues

I understand quite well that in most cases of M-S pain, you can easily identify the physical cause—an injury or accident—that triggered your pain; however, I believe everything in life happens for a reason and there are no accidents. Pain is a messenger, and it's in your life to teach you a valuable lesson about yourself.

I would strongly suggest using MMJ to heighten self-awareness and help you in this healing process to get high with an intention. For example, you can ask the question "What is this pain about? What do I have to learn from the pain?" You will invariably receive valuable input in the form of thoughts, visions, or messages that either directly or indirectly respond to the questions you've asked. It's helpful to have a journal in which to record this information. The process works similarly with meditation.

In addition to receiving input from your soul, higher self, and spirit guides through MMJ or meditation, I have found Louise Hay and her book *You Can Heal Your Life* to be a consistently reliable resource for helping to clarify the issues and the message of the chronic pain. Ms. Hay published this remarkable book in 1984, after healing herself from stage 4 ovarian cancer. I have continued using the book as a mind-body reference for more than thirty years, to help me and my patients better understand the mental, emotional, and spiritual causes of their pain and dis-ease. Once you have more clarity about the underlying source of your pain, it can facilitate your healing.

Each of the following physical problems is followed by the possible mental and emotional issues contributing to it, and then an *affirmation* that might help relieve the problem. This material is derived predominantly from Louise Hay.

> *Knees*: This pair is representative of stubborn ego and pride; inability to bend; fear; inflexibility; won't give in. Knee pain can also result from conflict between your authentic self and tribal teachings. "Tribal" refers to community—i.e., family, coworkers, religion. *I bend and flow with ease, and all is well.*

> *Neck*: This embodies a refusal to see other sides of a question; stubbornness; inflexibility. *It is with flexibility and ease that I see all sides of an issue. There are endless ways of doing and seeing things. I am safe.*

> *Shoulders*: These are meant to carry joy, not burdens. Shouldering too much responsibility; too many *shoulds*—universal or too much *shoulding* on yourself. *I am free to be joyous.*

> *Hips*: They are about fear of going forward in major decisions; nothing to move forward to; self-pity. *I am in perfect balance. I move forward in life with ease and with joy at every age.*

Ankles: This pair represents mobility and direction. *I move forward easily in life.*

Wrists: These represent movement and ease. *I handle all my experiences with wisdom, with love, and with ease.*

Patient Story—**Musculoskeletal Pain**

Brian R. is a twenty-six-year-old graduate student who badly fractured his right ankle (both tibia and fibula) in a skiing accident in February 2015. The surgical repair involved a metal plate and several screws, and resulted in chronic ankle pain with which he continues to suffer. Post-operatively he was prescribed Vicodin, but he was unable to maintain the mental clarity he needed for his PhD program in engineering, and he disliked the other side effects he experienced, such as constipation and nausea.

Within two to three weeks following his surgery, on the recommendation of his roommate, Brian began using marijuana for pain relief. It worked well enough for him to obtain an MMJ license.

Brian's orthopedist has told him he may have to live with some degree of pain for the rest of his life, and can only offer him opioids for pain relief. The pain is worse later in the day, when Brian rates it as a 5. MMJ has offered him relief though. He typically uses it when he gets home after class. Late afternoon he'll vaporize a hybrid, often Harlequin or a 60:40 or 70:30/indica strain, which almost immediately reduces his pain to a 1–2. He also uses tinctures, both 2:1 and 3:1/CBD:THC, with good results. Before bed he ingests indica edibles, which relieve the pain and help him get a good night's sleep, and be nearly pain-free to start the new day.

Chapter 12

Neuropathic (Nerve) Pain: Neuropathy, Shingles, Trigeminal Neuralgia, Complex Regional Pain Syndrome

Surrender

A ll of the diagnoses presented in this chapter involve the body's nervous system and are among the most painful of all the chronic pain conditions. Of the various tissues in the human body, nerves take longest to heal. Due to its severity and duration, nerve pain is often disabling and difficult to treat. It typically requires the use of opioids, gabapentin, or Lyrica to relieve the pain, but these often cause a host of unpleasant side effects.

Gabapentin, an anticonvulsant (antiseizure) drug, is commonly used for treating shingles, trigeminal neuralgia, and diabetic and peripheral neuropathy. However, it is often not well tolerated, with uncomfortable side effects including drowsiness, dizziness, loss of coordination, tiredness, blurred/double vision, unusual eye movements, and shaking (tremor). Lyrica, also an anticonvulsant, is frequently prescribed for treating shingles pain and diabetic neuropathy. It can cause drowsiness, dizziness, dry mouth, constipation, and blurred vision.

Fortunately, medical marijuana has proven to be highly effective for relieving nerve pain, regardless of its cause or severity. The MMJ recommendations that follow can be used to treat each of the conditions presented in this chapter.

MEDICAL MARIJUANA RECOMMENDATIONS FOR NERVE PAIN

If you are suffering from any of these four types of neuralgia (nerve pain), and you are in an acute phase, one in which your pain is consistently at a 6–7 or above (this is quite common with neuropathic pain), then please don't be concerned about relying too heavily on medical marijuana. For fifteen weeks, early in the course of living with shingles, my pain level varied from a minimum of 7–8 at the beginning, to a minimum of 5 toward the end of this nearly five-month ordeal (the acute phase), and I averaged between four and seven MMJ products per day.

When you are attempting to function and live your life as normally as possible in spite of unrelenting incapacitating pain, don't hesitate to use as much medical marijuana as you need to be reasonably comfortable. But please wait for at least one to two hours after taking an MMJ product (other than through inhalation) before determining if you need something more. Remember that tinctures take approximately thirty to forty-five minutes to begin working, with a peak effect beginning at about ninety minutes and lasting for up to five hours from the time it was administered. Edibles, ingested hash oil, tablets, capsules, or anything else that you take orally, can take up to two hours before the maximum peak effect begins, and this can last for six to seven hours from the time you swallowed the edible. I understand quite well your impatience and your discomfort, but my point here is to make sure you need something more before taking additional medicine. This way you can take the next product as the effect of the first one is beginning to wear off, with minimal overlap.

Although the products that are most effective for relieving pain contain moderate amounts of THC, you need not worry about "getting too high." It seems that when treating severe pain with products containing nearly equal amounts of CBD and THC, somehow either the CBD or the pain itself (or both) significantly reduce the psychoactive effect of the THC. It's definitely present but relatively mild.

You should also be aware that it is the psychoactive effect that contributes heavily to your pain relief. I've heard several patients tell me in almost the same words, "I'm not sure if the THC is doing anything directly to reduce the pain, but it sure takes my mind off it."

- Vaporize hash oil—either 1:1, 2:1, or 3:1/CBD:THC or Rick Simpson oil/Phoenix Tears. This seems to be the most effective method for relief of nerve pain.
- Ingest these same hash oils—start with a low dose (an amount equal to 1 short grain of rice) and gradually increase. Please note that the potency of hash oil varies from 600 to 900 mg per gram of oil, so the stronger the oil, the smaller the grain of rice. Eat with a fatty food.
- Vaporize hybrids—either 50:50 or 60:40/S:I, or 60:40/I:S, especially Harlequin (a 50:50 strain with high CBD).
- Dab a concentrate (shatter, wax, resin)—reserve this for only the most severe pain that is unresponsive to other methods. It should be used only as a last-resort treatment if all else has failed. WARNING: Dabbing on a daily basis, especially concentrates high in THC, may result in "burning out" your endocannabinoid receptors, rendering you unresponsive to any form of marijuana. The high-potency THC concentrates can also be addictive. These risks can be mitigated with the use of CBD:THC oils, which are more effective for pain relief. If the higher concentrates are needed, then use a vaporizer rather than a dab rig.
- Nasal spray—1:1/CBD:THC; CBD:THC:CBN, for pain and sleep. This is a new product and should be available by the latter part of 2017.
- Tinctures—1:1 or 2:1/CBD:THC; CBD:THC:CBN, for pain and sleep. With severe pain, tinctures are almost never sufficient by themselves, but do work quite well in combination with other delivery methods, such as the CBD capsules.
- CBD capsules or tincture—with less than 1 percent THC, 50–100 mg; use *in addition* to any of these MMJ recommendations. The CBD will enhance the analgesic and anti-inflammatory effect of the other options and help reduce anxiety and the psychoactive effect of THC. The less your anxiety, the lower your pain level.
- CBN capsules are helpful for both pain relief and sleep.

- Indica tablets, both swallowed (Stratos Sleep) and sublingual (Med-a-mints Indica)—excellent for pain and sleep. Stratos tablets are also available in 1:1/CBD:THC (for pain) and 15:1 (for sleep).
- SOS Pain sublingual tablets are also effective for nerve pain.
- Juice raw cannabis leaves. If that's not an option, use THCa, CBDa, and CBD tinctures as an alternative.
- Topicals—generalized (apply to wrist or ankle for rapid absorption) transdermal patches, especially 3:2/CBDa:THCa; THCa; 1:1/CBD:THC. CBN patches are excellent for both pain and sleep (and are not psychoactive). Also Mary's Medicinal's transdermal gel pens THC or CBD in combination with other delivery methods.
- Topicals—localized (apply to painful areas).
- Vaporize indica strains—70:30/I:S or above, for pain and sleep.
- Indica and hybrid edibles—gluten-free, without sugar or dairy; use indica for pain and sleep.

Keep in mind the *value of a good night's sleep* when treating severe pain. The less sleep you have, the greater your anxiety, which then typically causes more pain. Good quality sleep is also restorative and very helpful to the healing process of your damaged nerves.

NEUROPATHY

The nervous system is a complex network of nerves and cells that carry messages from the brain and spinal cord to various parts of the body. The nervous system includes both the central nervous system (brain and spinal cord) and peripheral nervous system (somatic and autonomic nervous systems).

Neuropathy is quite common, affecting more than 20 million Americans. It can occur at any age, but is more common among older adults. The term is used to describe a problem with the nerves, usually the peripheral nerves as opposed to the central nervous system. Neuropathy is seen with a number of different underlying medical conditions, such as physical trauma, repetitive injury, infection, metabolic problems, and exposure to toxins and some drugs. But it is most commonly associated with diabetes. In approximately 30 percent of patients with neuropathy, there is no known cause. This is called *idiopathic neuropathy*.

As with all of the neuropathic pain conditions presented in this chapter, as well as each of the chronic pain conditions described in this book, conventional medicine has no cure, only symptom relief. Therefore, the primary objective for both conventional and holistic medical treatment is to focus on the causes.

SHINGLES

Shingles is a viral infection that causes a painful rash. Although shingles can occur anywhere on your body, it most often appears as a single stripe of blisters that wraps around either the left or the right side of your torso.

Shingles is caused by the herpes zoster virus—the same virus that causes chicken pox. After you've had chicken pox, the virus lies inactive in nerve tissue near your spinal cord and brain. Years later, the virus may reactivate as shingles.

While it isn't a life-threatening condition, shingles can be extremely painful. (I describe my personal experience with shingles in the Introduction. It was the severity of the pain and its remarkable response to MMJ that inspired me to write this book.) Vaccines can help reduce the risk of shingles, while early treatment can help shorten a shingles infection and lessen the chance of post-herpetic neuralgia (pain lasting for longer than three months).

The signs and symptoms of shingles usually affect only a small section of one side of your body. These may include:

- Pain, burning, numbness or tingling—typically the first symptom
- Sensitivity to touch
- A red rash that begins a few days after the pain
- Fluid-filled blisters that break open and crust over
- Itching

Some people experience shingles pain without ever developing the rash.

TRIGEMINAL NEURALGIA

Trigeminal neuralgia (TN), also called *tic douloureux*, is a chronic pain condition that affects the trigeminal, or fifth cranial nerve, one of the most widely distributed nerves in the head. TN occurs most often in people over age fifty, although it can occur at any age, including infancy. The incidence of new cases is approximately twelve per one hundred thousand people per year, and it is more common in women than in men.

The typical or "classic" form of TN (Type 1) causes extreme, sporadic, sudden burning or shock-like facial pain that lasts anywhere from a few seconds to as long as two minutes per episode. These attacks can occur in quick succession, in volleys lasting as long as two hours. The "atypical" form of the disorder (Type 2) is characterized by a constant aching, burning, stabbing pain of somewhat lower intensity than Type 1. Both forms of pain may occur in the same person, sometimes at the same time. The intensity of pain can be physically and mentally incapacitating.

The trigeminal nerve is one of twelve pairs of nerves that are attached to the brain (cranial nerves). The nerve has three branches that conduct sensations from the upper, middle, and lower portions of the face, as well as the oral cavity, to the brain. The ophthalmic, or upper, branch supplies sensation to most of the scalp, forehead, and front of the head. The maxillary, or middle, branch stimulates the cheek, upper jaw, top lip, teeth and gums, and the side of the nose. The mandibular, or lower, branch conducts nerve impulses to the lower jaw, teeth and gums, and bottom lip. More than one nerve branch can be affected by TN.

TN is associated with a variety of conditions. It can be caused by a blood vessel pressing on the trigeminal nerve as it exits the brain stem. This compression causes wearing away or damage to the protective coating around the nerve (the myelin sheath). TN symptoms can also occur in people with multiple sclerosis (MS), a disease that also causes deterioration of the trigeminal nerve's myelin sheath. Rarely, symptoms of TN may be caused by nerve compression from a tumor or a tangle of arteries and veins called an arteriovenous malformation. Injury to the trigeminal nerve (perhaps the result of sinus surgery, oral surgery, stroke, or facial trauma) may also produce neuropathic facial pain.

The intense flashes of pain associated with Type 1 can be triggered by vibration or contact with the cheek (such as when shaving, washing the face, or applying makeup), brushing teeth, eating, drinking, talking, or being exposed to the wind. The pain may affect a small area of the face or may spread. Bouts of pain rarely occur at night, when the affected individual is sleeping.

TN is typified by attacks that stop for a period of time and then return, but the condition can be progressive. The attacks often worsen over time, with fewer and shorter pain-free periods before they recur. Eventually, the pain-free intervals disappear and medication to control the pain becomes less effective. Although not fatal, TN can be quite debilitating. Due to the intensity of the pain, some individuals may avoid daily activities or social contacts because they fear an impending attack.

Conventional treatment for TN includes medication and surgery. Anticonvulsant medicines, used to block nerve firing, are generally effective in treating TN1 but often less effective in TN2. Although these drugs, including carbamazepine, oxcarbazepine, and gabapentin, might be effective in relieving symptoms, many patients have difficulty tolerating their side effects. This is also true of the tricyclic antidepressants such as amitriptyline or nortriptyline, which can also be used to treat pain. Common analgesics and opioids are not usually helpful in treating the sharp, recurring pain caused by TN1, although some individuals with TN2 do respond to opioids. Eventually, if medication fails to relieve pain or produces intolerable side effects such as cognitive disturbances, memory loss, excess fatigue, bone marrow suppression, or allergy, then surgical treatment may be indicated. Since TN is a progressive disorder that often becomes resistant to medication over time, individuals often seek this surgical option.

COMPLEX REGIONAL PAIN SYNDROME (CRPS)

Complex regional pain syndrome, also known as reflex sympathetic dystrophy syndrome (RSD), is described in the medical literature as *chronic arm or leg pain developing after injury, surgery, stroke, or heart attack*. It's rare, with fewer than two hundred thousand U.S. cases per year, and is considered incurable, but treatment may help. CRPS is believed to be caused by damage to, or malfunction of, the peripheral and central nervous systems. The syndrome is characterized by prolonged or excessive pain, mild or dramatic changes in skin color and temperature, and/or swelling in the affected area. It can last for years or a lifetime, and is among the most debilitating of all chronic pain conditions. I have seen several patients suffering with CRPS, and it is devastating.

CRPS symptoms vary in severity and duration. Studies of the incidence and prevalence of the disease show that most cases are mild and individuals recover gradually with time. In more severe cases, individuals may not recover and may have long-term disability.

Anyone can get CRPS. It can strike at any age and affects both men and women, although it is much more common in women. The average age of affected individuals is about forty, and CRPS is rare in the elderly. Children do not get it before age five and only very rarely before age ten, but it is not uncommon in teenagers.

The key symptom is prolonged pain that may be constant and, in some people, extremely uncomfortable or severe. The pain may feel like a burning or "pins and needles" sensation, or as if someone is squeezing the affected limb. The pain may spread to include the entire arm or leg, even though the precipitating injury might have been only to a finger or toe. Pain can sometimes even travel to the opposite extremity. There is often increased sensitivity in the affected area, such that even light touch or contact is painful (called *allodynia*).

People with CRPS also experience constant or intermittent changes in skin temperature and color, and swelling of the affected limb. This is due to abnormal microcirculation caused by damage to the nerves controlling blood flow and temperature. An affected arm or leg may feel warmer or cooler compared to the opposite limb. The skin on the affected limb may change color, becoming blotchy, blue, purple, pale, or red.

In more than 90 percent of cases, the condition is triggered by a clear history of trauma or injury. The most common triggers are fractures, sprains/strains, soft tissue injury (such as burns, cuts, or bruises), limb immobilization (such as being in a cast), or damage from surgical or medical procedures (such as needlestick). CRPS represents an abnormal response that magnifies the effects of the injury. In this respect it is like an allergy. Some people respond excessively to a trigger that causes no problem for other people.

HOLISTIC MEDICAL TREATMENT AND PREVENTION PROGRAM FOR NEUROPATHIC PAIN

Risk Factors and Causes

- *Medication*—Nearly forty drugs are known to cause neuropathy.
- *Diabetes*—The most common cause of chronic peripheral neuropathy (high blood sugar levels in people with poorly controlled diabetes damage nerves).
- *B12 or folate vitamin deficiencies*—can cause nerve damage and peripheral neuropathy.
- *Poisons (toxins)*—Insecticides and solvents can cause peripheral nerve damage.
- *Cancers*—Peripheral neuropathy can occur in people with some cancers; e.g., lymphoma and multiple myeloma.
- *Alcohol excess*—High alcohol levels in the body cause nerve damage.
- *Chronic kidney disease*—If the kidneys are not functioning normally, an imbalance of salts and chemicals can cause peripheral neuropathy.
- *Chronic liver disease*.
- *Injuries*—Broken bones and tight plaster casts can put pressure directly on the nerves, and this can also cause CRPS.
- *Infections*—Damage can be caused to peripheral nerves by some infections, including shingles, HIV infection, and Lyme disease.
- *Guillain-Barré syndrome*—the name given to a specific type of peripheral neuropathy triggered by infection.

Physical Health Recommendations

Remove the cause: Stop the medication, eliminate the toxin, control the diabetes, treat the infection.

Diet

Follow the anti-inflammatory diet in Chapter 5. Since neuropathic pain often involves some degree of dysfunction or damage to the myelin sheath surrounding nerve cells (neurons), nutrients that help repair the myelin (composed of 70 percent fat) will help to heal the painful nerves. These foods are relatively high in the amino acids choline and inositol, and include avocados, olive oil, fish, raw nuts, cocoa, whole grains, legumes, spinach (raw), beans, eggs, and beef. Choline assists in preventing fatty deposits from forming in the body. Inositol supports a healthy nervous system by helping to create serotonin. These two amino acids combine to produce lecithin, which reduces unhealthy fats that are known to prevent myelin sheath repair.

Especially with shingles, *foods high in the amino acid arginine should be avoided*. These include seafood, liver, seeds (sesame, sunflower, pumpkin), soy, fish, turkey, pork, game meat, beef, spinach, and most common nuts (including almonds, brazil nuts, hazelnuts, macadamia nuts, pine nuts, pistachios, and walnuts). *Foods high in the amino acid lysine* can help prevent recurrence of shingles outbreaks. These include legumes, eggs, yogurt, fish (including salmon and tuna), and chicken.

Vitamins, Minerals, and Supplements

NOTE: Supplements used for diminishing nerve pain may take three to twelve months to have a noticeable therapeutic effect.

- *PhosphaLine* (Xymogen): PhosphaLine provides 2.7 gm of pure polyenylphosphatidylcholine (PPC) per serving plus the highest concentrated source of 1,2 DLPC (dilinoleoylphosphatidylcholine). *Choline, and specifically phosphatidylcholine, is a major component of the myelin sheath.* Unlike most other phosphatidylcholine products on the market, aside from PPC and DLPC, PhosphaLine contains no other phospholipids, which may compete for absorption. Studies suggest that PPC ingestion increases choline levels in the blood and brain and supports acetylcholine synthesis for healthy neuronal and cell function. Daily supplementation of PPC may help maintain healthy brain and liver function, and provide gastric mucosal protection. Recommended dosage is 2 to 3 softgels daily with food.
- *Inositol*: Take up to 1,000 mg daily; it can also be found in nuts, vegetables, grains, soy, and bananas.

- *B-Activ* (Xymogen): This is an exceptional blend of methylated B vitamins. The recommended dosage is 1 tablet two times daily with food. Both B1 (thiamine) and B12 are components of the myelin sheath. B1 can also be obtained by eating rice, spinach, lentils, and pork. Foods rich in B vitamins include whole grains and dairy products. High-dose (5 mg) vitamin B12 injections can sometimes be helpful for relieving shingles pain, and possibly help some people with neuropathy. High-dose combinations of B12 and folate are available from health professionals.

- *Omega-3 fatty acids* (OmegaGenics EPA-DHA 720 from Metagenics): 1 capsule three times daily with food. Foods high in omega-3s include flaxseeds, fish oils, pumpkin and chia seeds, salmon and other deep-sea fish, walnuts, and kidney beans. *Oleic acid* is also a major component of the fatty myelin sheath, and can be found in the following foods: olive oil, avocados, and nuts.

- *ALAmax CR* (Xymogen): Timed-released alpha-lipoic acid in a high dose has been shown to potentially reduce peripheral neuropathy, especially in diabetic patients. ALAmax CR delivers 600 mg of timed-released alpha-lipoic acid. The recommended dosage is 1 capsule thirty minutes before breakfast and 1 capsule thirty minutes before dinner. It may take a few months before you notice any difference. Intravenous alpha-lipoic acid administered on a daily basis while gradually increasing the dose over a two-week period has been shown to help some patients with peripheral neuropathy.

- *Vitamin D*: A *dosage* of 2,000 units daily for three months was shown to decrease diabetic neuropathy pain by 47 percent. I recommend testing your vitamin D level (blood test). The goal is to maintain it around 80. You may need more additional Vitamin D than 2,000 units, but only increase the dose with professional supervision.

- *Acetyl-L-carnitine*: This has been shown to help some patients with diabetic neuropathy. The recommended dosage is 1,000 mg twice daily between meals.

- *Copper*: Helps to create an enzyme essential to lipid development. Lipids are needed for regeneration of the myelin sheath. Copper is found in lentils, almonds, pumpkin seeds, semisweet chocolate, oregano, and thyme. A health professional trained in Functional Medicine can measure your copper levels.

- *Alpha-GPC (L-Alpha Glycerylphosphorylcholine)*: This is another very stable and rapidly available form of choline found in the brain and in the myelin sheath. It has been shown to protect and repair damaged brain cells. The recommended dosage is 600–1,200 mg per day.
- *L-lysine and Vitamin C*: These can accelerate the healing process from shingles and reduce the risk of further outbreaks. I recommend 1,500 mg per day of L-lysine and 6,000–10,000 mg per day of vitamin C (as Ester-C). High-dose (50,000 mg) IV vitamin C can also be helpful.

Other Self-Care Techniques

Low-impact exercise, yoga, creative visualization, aroma therapy, and meditation are all useful in promoting well-being, and as a result help to relieve neuropathic pain.

Professional Care Therapies

Acupuncture, *aromatherapy*, *chiropractic*, and other types of *bodywork*; *biofeedback* and *relaxation techniques*; and especially *energy medicine* techniques, such as *Healing Touch*, can be helpful for treating each of the neuropathic pain conditions. As a certified Healing Touch practitioner, I've been amazed at the effectiveness of this modality for treating a wide variety of chronic pain conditions.

There have also been reports that injections of botulinum toxin, to block the activity of sensory nerves, offers modest pain relief to some sufferers of trigeminal neuralgia.

Chronic neuropathic pain can be very isolating and is frequently associated with profound psychological symptoms for affected individuals and their families. People with this level of disabling pain may develop depression, anxiety, posttraumatic stress disorder, and sleep disorders, all of which heighten the perception of pain and make rehabilitation efforts more difficult. *Psychotherapy* or supportive counseling can be beneficial for many of these patients. I recommend a cognitive, behavioral, or spiritual psychotherapist, rather than a psychiatrist, since the latter are generally far more focused on drug therapy than counseling. Treating these secondary conditions with psychotherapy is important for helping people cope and recover from chronic neuropathic pain.

The Issues in Your Tissues

As with all chronic pain conditions, there are several potentially life-changing lessons inherent in your dis-ease. As I mentioned in the Introduction, for me the primary message of shingles was *surrender*. When dealing with disabling pain, you really have no choice but to let go of trying to control your life. You feel helpless, hopeless, and powerless. And it is blatantly obvious that you're *not* in control.

With pain of this severity, you have the opportunity to build greater faith and trust that this condition has happened to you for a reason, one that will ultimately benefit you and change your life for the better. I believe that my soul chose my life's experiences prior to birth, and my life is unfolding just as it needs to in order to fulfill my purpose and greatest potential.

Shingles was possibly the greatest physical and emotional challenge I've ever faced, but at this point I'm quite sure I would not be writing this book had it not been for this horrendous virus and the relief I was provided by medical marijuana. And in spite of the thousands of patients I've seen who have been able to live reasonably well with chronic pain as a result of using MMJ, I doubt I would have been as passionate a proponent of this remarkable medicine had I not personally endured the pain of post-herpetic neuralgia.

Admittedly surrender and letting go of trying to control is a difficult lesson to learn for those of us who feel we need a large measure of control in order to feel safe, be successful, or to even survive in a hostile world. But as with every chronic pain condition, there are multiple lessons.

The issues in your tissues that have the strongest association with your physical pain can reliably be identified by the anatomical location of the pain and the chakra to which that location is most closely related. The neuropathic pain conditions (or any neurological dysfunction) described in this chapter—neuropathy, trigeminal neuralgia, CRPS, and shingles—are all associated with the sixth or brow chakra. At the top of the list of this chakra's mental/emotional issues is *self-evaluation*—i.e., being highly self-critical and too hard on yourself (*not loving yourself*). The other issues contributing to your physical pain may be: *feelings of inadequacy, truth, intellectual abilities, openness to the ideas of others, ability to learn from experience,* and *emotional intelligence.*

The issues for neuropathy, CRPS, and shingles sufferers whose pain is in a location other than the face and head may also include those associated with the closest chakra. In my case, the rash and pain extended across my abdomen and were related to the third chakra. The primary issues there are: *trust, power and control, sensitivity to criticism, fear and intimidation, self-esteem, self-respect, care of oneself and others,* and *responsibility for making decisions.*

Patient Story—**Neuropathy**

Donna B. is a sixty-one-year-old with a stressful job as a child support enforcer and a twelve-year history of neuropathy in both legs. It affects her feet, ankles, and legs, extending upward to just below her knees. The pain is constant at a level of 4–5, but is worse with increased stress. She does not have diabetes and the cause of her pain is unknown.

Throughout the course of the neuropathy she has relied on marijuana for relief. She was originally prescribed gabapentin but did not like the side effects. She found that the marijuana she obtained "off the street" (nearly all of which was a sativa or high-THC strain) was quite effective. After MMJ became available, and for the past seven years, she's been smoking indica strains on a daily basis after work. She rotates different indicas every few days, and usually has three or four different strains available to avoid developing a tolerance. It nearly always reduces the pain to a 2–3, in addition to significantly relieving her stress and helping her sleep. During workdays, she applies the topical MMJ cream Apothecanna Extra Strength to her legs. She says it helps, but not nearly as much as smoking indica.

Patient Story—**Trigeminal Neuralgia**

Marilyn F. is fifty-eight years old, unemployed, and on disability as a result of the trigeminal neuralgia that began five years ago. Her medical treatment started with Tegretol, which was moderately effective for relieving the pain when taken in high doses, but caused her to break out in "huge hives," which she scratched until she bled. That was followed by Neurontin, which caused a host of severe side effects—including weight gain, vision loss, kidney damage, and a speech impediment—and *no* pain relief. She suffered with these for two years, along with suicidal thoughts on a daily basis. She then had two surgical procedures, the first of which relieved her pain for seven months and the second of which for approximately one year.

Rather than have additional risky brain surgery, offering only temporary relief, she obtained an MMJ license, began growing her own plants, and started making Phoenix Tears (Rick Simpson Oil). She's been ingesting the oil two to three times daily (in amounts that vary from one to two grains of rice), and her pain level while using it is reduced to a 2–3. Without it, her pain was a consistent 9–10, with twenty to thirty attacks daily, and these attacks would leave her unable to speak, smile, laugh, eat, or drink. She was essentially incapacitated, but now the MMJ in her words "allows me to have a life." There are times when she has no pain at all.

Patient Story—CRPS

In 2001, at the age of twenty-four, Beth C. was in good health with no physical pain or significant emotional stress. She was physically active and either hiked or walked daily. According to her, "life was fine."

Then, in an instant, her life changed dramatically, when she rolled her SUV down a hill, flipped five times over a highway exit and landed right side up. She had fallen asleep on her way to work at 8:30 am. She lost all of her skin from her ankles down to her toes on both legs. She had apparently walked through a foot of snow while waiting for help.

She was admitted into a hospital with severe frostbite, a badly broken left ankle, and a seriously sprained right ankle. The physicians waited seventy-two hours before performing surgery on the ankle, in order to first determine whether they could save her toes. They decided to keep all ten toes. The surgical procedure resulted in a six-inch plate inserted in Beth's left ankle. She was in the hospital for more than a week, then transported to a rehabilitation facility for three and a half weeks.

There she began relearning to walk, which took approximately eight months, during which time she regrew the skin on both ankles and feet. Also during this time the pain *worsened*. Her doctors reassured her that it would go away, but each month it got worse.

Her life, as she described it, "was pretty bad; only doctors, pain and more problems. I tried water therapy, land therapy, exercises, stretches, but nothing helped."

The excruciating pain persisted. The injury had left her with chronic severe pain around the clock; leg soreness; severe leg cramping in her calves; constant aching legs with intermittent shooting and dull pain in both legs and ankles; stiffness in both ankles; severe back pain; neck pain; shoulder pain; and no sleep. Even a mild breeze of air would make her body hurt.

She had "no life left." She could no longer walk, sit, stand, or sleep without pain. Her pain level was a 10 every day and all day. She had severe restless leg syndrome, and couldn't sleep much at all. She would toss and turn for hours, with excruciating pain and leg soreness. The bedsheet would create more pain just by lying on top of her legs. She slept with multiple pillows at night lifting her legs and separating them so they wouldn't touch. She could no longer drive a car because the back pain was so horrible. She could no longer work, sit in a chair, watch TV, see friends, or even leave her house.

The narcotic medications she was prescribed would help for a short time, but her condition continued to worsen. She was also taking a variety of drugs for neuralgia (nerve pain), including gabapentin and Lyrica, in addition to muscle relaxants. None of the medications made a significant difference in her overall condition. They would help to a minimal extent when she increased the dosage or changed to a new medication, but the beneficial effects lasted for only a few months.

In 2006, she was finally diagnosed with complex regional pain syndrome (CRPS) or reflex sympathetic dystrophy syndrome (RSD). The diagnosis was made at Beth Israel Hospital in New York City, considered one of the region's top medical centers.

Unfortunately, having a definitive diagnosis had no positive impact on Beth's condition. She was still severely disabled. It had been several years of struggle with severe insomnia as well as nearly a 100 percent memory loss as a result of the medications. She was unable to remember things from two minutes earlier. The depression worsened, accompanied by suicidal thoughts and extreme anxiety. Severe anxiety attacks were more frequent and occasionally required a visit to an emergency room. During this period, she was also traveling monthly into New York City for a spinal injection and a visit to a psychiatrist, who prescribed several antidepressants and antianxiety medications. She was also prescribed drugs for sleep.

A recreational user of cannabis prior to the accident (she also used it to relieve anxiety), Beth started to smoke it much more frequently after her accident. She was having difficulty with stomachaches from all the medications, especially those with aspirin, acetaminophen, and added filler. Cannabis was the only effective way to settle her stomach. She also found that it helped to relieve her overall pain, muscle aches, and anxiety.

However, it was extremely difficult for her to medicate herself with marijuana in a state where it was illegal. In spite of having to rely on whatever strain she could find (usually high-THC sativa, which is not as effective for pain as the high-CBD strains), and being drug-screened monthly, she continued to use cannabis because of its beneficial effects on her condition. Every month she experienced the stress of being tested and not knowing if she was going to lose her doctor and be treated differently as a marijuana user.

In April of 2013, no longer able to afford medical insurance, grieving the recent loss of her father, and the divorce from her husband, she decided to stop seeing her doctors, stopped all of her medications, and moved to Colorado. These major changes took a toll on her, both physically and emotionally. But she believed that having legal access to medical marijuana in Colorado would be worth it.

She currently uses medical marijuana daily as her *only medication*. It not only keeps her feeling comfortable, but *her disease has been in remission since she moved to Colorado.*

The medical marijuana also controls Beth's anxiety, which decreases her pain. She occasionally has minimal pain with excessive physical activity, but "When I use the medicine [cannabis] it alleviates most of my symptoms instantly."

Since moving to Colorado, she has essentially created a new life. She developed a much more positive attitude and decided to "make every day a great day." She does yoga regularly, and takes her new dog for hikes and walks daily. After two months in Colorado she met her future husband while dancing at a concert. Although music had been a passion of hers before the accident, she hadn't attended a concert or danced in over ten years. Her passion for music, dancing, and a love life have all been rekindled. She remarried in August 2015.

Chapter 13

Dysmenorrhea (Menstrual Pain)

A Lesson in Self-Love

Dysmenorrhea is a condition in which women experience pain during menstruation. The pain occurs during the ovulatory cycle and is caused by excess production of prostaglandins. Prostaglandins are hormone-like complex fatty acids that belong to the family of eicosanoids. Eicosanoids are present in tissues throughout the body and are involved in inflammation. They also have other functions, including smooth muscle contractility, blood clotting, vascular dilation, and immunity.

The primary types of prostaglandins are *anti-inflammatory prostaglandins* (PGE1 and PGE3), which decrease inflammation, and *pro-inflammatory prostaglandins* (PGE2 and PGF2 alpha), which cause uterine contraction. When there is an imbalance and an increased production of PGE2 in the uterus, dysmenorrhea is the result.

The pro-inflammatory prostaglandins have a stimulating effect on the uterus. The endometrium (uterine lining normally shed during the bleeding phase) secretes excess prostaglandin, which causes the smooth muscle of the uterus to contract, leading to cramping and pain. In some cases the constriction and tightening of the uterine muscle are so severe that blood circulation and oxygen to the uterine muscle is severely diminished. Metabolic waste products like carbon dioxide and lactic acid accumulate and tend to make the pain worse.

An excessive release of pro-inflammatory prostaglandins during the sloughing of the endometrium is a popular and valid explanation for this painful condition. But there is another theory that states that dysmenorrhea is an inflammatory disorder due to an imbalance of fats (phospholipids) in the cell membranes throughout the body. Dietary fats are broken down into prostaglandins through a series of metabolic steps. This involves optimal enzyme conversion to better shunt certain fats toward PGE1 and PGE3 (anti-inflammatory) and away from PGE2 (pro-inflammatory). In some cases these enzymes do not work optimally due to aging, family history (genetics), environmental toxins, cigarette smoking, disease, or vitamin and mineral deficiencies.

It is estimated that as many as 30 to 50 percent of women suffer from pain during menstruation. However, this is a conservative figure, since most women don't seek medical treatment for dysmenorrhea.

There are two classifications of dysmenorrhea—primary (by far, the most common) and secondary. *Primary dysmenorrhea* occurs when the pain itself is the main problem. At least 10 percent of younger women (teens and early twenties) have symptoms so severe that they cannot go to school, work, or participate in normal activities. Some women also experience low back pain, pinching and pain sensations in the inner thighs, as well as many premenstrual symptoms (breast tenderness, weight gain, headaches, bloating, and irritability). Women in their thirties and forties tend to have more severe cases of dysmenorrhea, especially if they have an excess estrogen imbalance.

Secondary dysmenorrhea is menstrual pain caused by an underlying pathological factor, such as endometriosis, pelvic inflammatory disease, or a congenital deformity.

MEDICAL MARIJUANA RECOMMENDATIONS FOR DYSMENORRHEA

I have seen a number of women who have had excellent results treating their menstrual pain with MMJ. Their dysmenorrhea is well controlled using indica or high-CBD products, especially CBD Cheeba Chews. These are edibles lasting for six to eight hours that allow you to function well throughout most of the day without pain, drowsiness, or getting high at work or school. CBD, as an analgesic, anti-inflammatory, and muscle relaxant without the psychoactive effect, is an ideal choice for women suffering with severe menstrual pain.

In addition to edibles, high-CBD tinctures and hash oils (ingested), both with low amounts of THC, are also effective, with minimal if any psychoactivity.

For topicals, I highly recommend Mary Jane's Medicinals Cannabis Infused Massage Oil, which is high in both THC and CBD. It deeply penetrates the uterine muscle, and patients report that it creates a sensation of "dissolving the cramps away."

I've also heard from several patients that the topical cream Apothecanna Extra Strength works well for less severe cramps. It's a good choice for more mild pain while at work or school.

Another recent addition to the MMJ options for treating menstrual pain are the Foria Relief vaginal suppositories (high CBD/low THC). Their availability in dispensaries is still limited, but the few patients I've seen who have used them were extremely pleased with the results.

THCa tincture as a strong anti-inflammatory can provide considerable relief and prevention when taken consistently throughout menstruation.

I would also highly recommend medicated bath products during menstruation. Dixie THC Infused Bath Soak (bath salts) and Mary Jane's Medicinals Heavenly Hash Bath (bath tea bag) are both excellent options for providing relief of severe menstrual pain.

Transdermal patches are also effective for daytime use in relieving menstrual pain. Nearly all the available patches can be beneficial, depending on the most prominent symptoms: CBD, 1:1/CBD:THC, THCa, THC-indica, THC-sativa, and CBN.

HOLISTIC MEDICAL TREATMENT AND PREVENTION PROGRAM FOR DYSMENORRHEA

Risk Factors and Causes

- *Poor diet*—one of the primary risk factors for dysmenorrhea. *Nutrient deficiency* is a common contributing factor. The most common depleted nutrients are antioxidants and magnesium. An excess amount of unhealthy fats (hydrogenated and trans-fatty acids) also contribute to menstrual pain.

- *Food allergies*—can lead to inflammation in the gut, known as "leaky gut," which increases permeability of the intestinal wall. Food allergies make the intestine a conducive environment for pathogens (parasites, bacteria, yeast overgrowth) to grow, which are also strong contributors to dysmenorrhea, especially if constipation is involved.
- *Hormone imbalance*—Hormones are metabolized through the liver. If the liver is congested due to gastrointestinal problems, then hormones can become imbalanced and cause estrogen dominance and adrenal insufficiency. If the thyroid gland is not functioning optimally, then this too can exacerbate painful menstruation.
- *Stress*—contributes to dysmenorrhea by raising cortisol and causing excess estrogen and low levels of progesterone.

NOTE: The conventional medical treatment of choice for most women with dysmenorrhea is nonsteroidal anti-inflammatory drugs (NSAIDS), such as ibuprofen. The overuse of these drugs can cause liver toxicity, in addition to decreasing blood flow to the kidneys.

Physical Health Recommendations

Diet

Prostaglandins are made from fatty acids. By modifying the types of fats you consume in your diet, you can manipulate your prostaglandin levels in favor of more anti-inflammatory prostaglandins (PGE1 and PGE3), which decrease inflammation and produce less pro-inflammatory prostaglandins (PGE2). The foods primarily responsible for increasing PGE2 contain *omega-6 fatty acids*. The precursor to PGE2 is an omega-6 fat known as arachidonic acid (AA). The body produces this AA naturally, but it also comes from foods.

Your goal is to *eliminate or significantly reduce rich dietary sources of AA*, such as: egg yolks, beef, lamb, and high-fat dairy products. The production of AA in the body also increases whenever you consume sugar or other high-glycemic foods, such as white bread, white potatoes, and bananas. Eating more fresh fruits and vegetables and whole grains, and moderate amounts of proteins such as seafood and soy (non-GMO), will reduce AA production.

The anti-inflammatory prostaglandins (PGE1 and PGE3) come from the fatty acid eicosapentaenoic (EPA). Cold-water fish (cod, tuna, herring, salmon, sardines, and mackerel) and fish oils will raise EPA levels. The two main fatty acids found in fish oil are EPA and DHA. Vegetarians can indirectly produce EPA from omega-3 fats found in walnuts and flax.

Another dietary recommendation is to reduce hydrogenated and trans-fatty acids.

Lowering alcohol and sugars helps to lower insulin as well as balance blood sugars and lower cholesterol levels.

Vitamins, Minerals, and Supplements

- *Fatty acids*: With dysmenorrhea, women typically need 3,000–5,000 mg of combined EPA/DHA daily. Healthy women, without menstrual pain, should take 1,100 mg daily.
- *Vitamin E*: 200–400 IU as d-alpha tocopherol with mixed tocopherols is recommended. Vitamin E releases endorphins, which block pain, within fifteen minutes after taking it.
- *Niacin*: 100 mg twice daily starting seven days before menstruation, then every two to three hours during cramping. It may cause flushing as the dose increases. It is also more effective when combined with vitamin C.
- *B6 and magnesium*: the cofactors that help enzymes work effectively in the production of anti-inflammatory prostaglandins. Magnesium is a smooth muscle relaxant, dilates pelvic blood vessels, and inhibits the production of the pro-inflammatory prostaglandins PGE2 and PGF2 alpha. Taking magnesium with B6 boosts its effectiveness. It's recommended to start with 300 mg of magnesium and increase until you have a soft stool. The dose for B6 is 100 mg taken in a B-complex supplement. Magnesium and B vitamins can also be infused intravenously prior to or during menstrual pain. This can both prevent and effectively relieve pain very quickly.
- *Curcumin*: very effective in reducing inflammation. The recommended dosage is 400 mg three times per day.
- *Ginger powder capsules*: Take 750–2,000 mg per day for the first three to four days of the menstrual cycle. Ginger root reduces prostaglandin production and reduces pain and inflammation.

Other Self-Care Techniques

1. *Avoid* food allergens and constipation.
2. *Stress reduction* and *exercise* help reduce hormone imbalance.

Professional Care Therapies

I recommend *colon cleansing* (colonics/colon hydrotherapy) and *liver detoxing* under professional supervision, *acupuncture*, and *psychotherapy/counseling* (especially if you relate to the description in "The Issues in Your Tissues" below).

The Issues in Your Tissues

Painful menstruation is often associated with a dislike of one's body. Lack of self-acceptance and self-love are typically accompanied by anger with oneself. This emotional profile may have begun in a family in which a woman felt devalued, denigrated, and powerless. This was then transformed into a strong dislike of herself and of being a woman.

Louise Hay, in *You Can Heal Your Life*, describes the probable emotional cause of menstrual problems as "rejection of one's femininity; guilt; fear; belief that the genitals are sinful or dirty." The affirmation she recommends: *I accept my full power as a woman and accept all of my bodily processes as normal and natural. I love and approve of myself.*

Patient Story—**Dysmenorrhea**

Rachel F. is a thirty-four-year-old graduate student who has been suffering with what she describes as "extreme and nearly incapacitating menstrual cramps" since high school. She reports having had to frequently stay home from school or work when the pain was most acute. She also has had a problem with severe anxiety.

Since she began using medical marijuana about four years ago, her symptoms, both the cramps and the anxiety, have significantly improved. She has had the greatest benefit from vaporizing Harlequin and other high-CBD and indica strains, in addition to CBD Cheeba Chews (an edible). She's also noticed some moderate improvement from applying the topical cream Apothecanna Extra Strength to her lower abdomen above her uterus, even without doing any of the other MMJ products.

When I mentioned the "issues in your tissues" that are typically present in women with dysmenorrhea, she became somewhat animated and replied, "Wow, that describes me perfectly!"

Chapter 14

Alleviating Cancer Pain

Grieve Your Loss

C ancer is officially the second leading cause of death in the U.S., killing approximately 500,000 people (more than 20 percent of all deaths) every year. Although the 2004 study "Death by Medicine" was never published in a medical journal, it ranks cancer as the third leading cause of death behind medical treatment and heart disease. Since 1958, the incidence of cancer in men has increased 55 percent. The curve of cancer incidence rises steeply after the age of sixty. A number of potential contributing causes have fueled the increase.

Cancer is a distorted, wild, uncontrolled growth of portions of body tissues or organs in which cells multiply rapidly without restraint, producing a family of descendants that invade and destroy the structure and function of adjacent normal tissues in the organ where the tumor originated. Cancerous cells can also travel through the bloodstream or lymph channels to lodge elsewhere in the body, starting new growths (metastases) and compromising the function of organs to which the cells spread.

The initial phase of cancerous growth is triggered by a distortion in the DNA command apparatus of the nucleus of body cells. Many researchers believe that human beings in a single lifetime experience cancer many times and that on most occasions the chemical and cellular immune defenses defeat the new growth so quickly that no symptoms ever make themselves known. It is recommended that we pay more attention to the state of our immune system, which for a variety of reasons occasionally fails to recognize and eliminate these early growths before they can become a threat. Damage to DNA in cell nuclei from free radical proliferation appears to play a key role in the initiation and growth of cancer.

Although this chapter's focus is on relieving cancer pain, effective treatment of the cancer itself will usually result in a reduction of pain. For this reason I will address, to a limited extent, cancer treatment in both the MMJ and HMTP sections.

Most cancer pain is caused by the tumor pressing on bones, nerves, or other organs in your body. Sometimes pain is related to cancer treatment, such as surgery, chemotherapy, or radiation. For example, some chemotherapy drugs can cause numbness and tingling in your hands and feet or a burning sensation at the place where they are injected. Radiation can also cause pain as a result of inflammation of the surrounding normal tissue.

Chronic pain associated with cancer is also caused by changes to nerves, which may occur due to the cancer pressing on the nerves, or due to chemicals produced by a tumor.

MEDICAL MARIJUANA RECOMMENDATIONS FOR CANCER PAIN

The recommendations for alleviating cancer *pain* overlap with the recommendations for treating the cancer itself. Much of the research for treating cancer with cannabis comes from Israel and to a lesser extent from Spain. Both THC and CBD have been shown to have cancer cell–killing properties. The combination of both cannabinoids into a substance called *Rick Simpson Oil (RSO)* or *Phoenix Tears* (see Chapter 4) is widely considered to be the single most effective MMJ product for *treating cancer*. It is also an excellent combination for *pain relief*.

This thick, dark brown, sticky hash oil is most often dispensed in a syringe, but is also available in capsules and rectal suppositories. The recommended dose is an amount approximately the size of one grain of rice. I suggest starting with less if you are someone who is particularly sensitive to THC (or pharmaceutical drugs). Depending on who makes it, there is a wide range of RSO composition with respect to the amount of THC. The most therapeutic for cancer seem to be those that have approximately 10 percent or more of THC. The THC is nearly always present in greater amounts than CBD, and it will therefore have a fairly strong psychoactive effect. For some cancer patients, this is a significant liability of RSO. However, this effect can possibly be minimized by using the rectal suppositories. To learn more about this method of administration, visit http://phoenixtears.ca/dosage-information/.

I recommend *ingesting* RSO or the rectal suppositories rather than vaporizing, since its duration of action is roughly twice as long when ingested (six to eight hours). This amount (one grain of rice) should be ingested twice a day. In addition, vaporizing the oil requires a vaporizer that accommodates oil which requires much higher temperature than flower (440 degrees Fahrenheit versus 375). It is therefore much more harsh on the mucous membrane lining the respiratory tract.

I suggest ingesting the oil with a fatty food—e.g., avocado or peanut butter—since marijuana is fat-soluble and this will allow for more rapid absorption, sometimes as quickly as thirty to forty-five minutes. The suppositories have an even more rapid onset—ten to fifteen minutes. Otherwise it might take one to even two hours before you feel a strong therapeutic effect. Since the oil is so sticky, it helps to push it out of the syringe onto a relatively hard surface, such as a cracker, and then you can scrape off the remaining oil at the opening of the syringe onto the cracker. After the dose of oil has been dispensed, then add your fatty food, and eat the whole thing. I don't recommend eating a sizable meal along with the oil, unless it's an especially fatty meal. A big meal will significantly delay the onset of the hash oil effect. For fastest absorption an empty stomach (other than the fatty food) is best.

If your focus is greater on treating the pain than on the cancer itself, in addition to RSO, the MMJ recommendations are essentially the same as those for musculoskeletal pain (Chapter 11) and osteoarthritis pain (Chapter 6), with the exception of a greater emphasis on treating inflammation for those suffering with arthritis. Most people's cancer pain has an inflammatory component, but it is not quite as severe as it is with arthritis.

- Topicals—localized (apply to painful area), especially Apothecanna Extra Strength or Mary's Medicinals CBC.
- Topicals—generalized (apply to wrist or ankle for rapid absorption) transdermal patches, especially 1:1/CBD:THC, 3:2/CBDa:THCa, THCa; also Mary's Medicinals transdermal gel pens, CBD, THC, or CBN.
- Vaporizing high-CBD strains of flower—especially Harlequin (a 50:50/S:I hybrid), Lucy (a 70:30/I:S indica), Cannatonic (a 50:50 hybrid), or other hybrids (either 50:50, 60:40/S:I, or 60:40/I:S).
- High-CBD tinctures—1:1, 2:1, or 3:1/CBD:THC.
- High-CBD hash oil—1:1, 3:1, or 6:1/CBD:THC.
- Juicing raw cannabis leaves.
- Indica strains of flower—with an I:S of 70:30 or above (also good for sleep).
- Indica and hybrid edibles—gluten-free, without sugar or dairy (also good for sleep).
- Any strain or MMJ product containing CBG.

NOTE: Avoid sativa strains above 60:40/S:I and high-THC products. Although THC has both analgesic and anti-inflammatory properties, it can also increase anxiety, which has the potential to increase pain.

HOLISTIC MEDICAL TREATMENT AND PREVENTION PROGRAM FOR CANCER PAIN

Types and Causes

- *Nerve pain*—caused by pressure from the tumor on nerves or the spinal cord, or by damage to nerves. This is also neuropathic pain (see Chapter 12). People often describe nerve pain as burning, shooting, tingling, or as a feeling of something crawling under their skin. It can be difficult to describe exactly how it feels, and it is often more difficult to treat than other types of pain.

    Some people have long-term nerve pain after surgery. Nerves may be cut during an operation, and they take a long time to heal because they grow very slowly. Some people may have pain around their scar for two years or more after their surgery, but it eventually goes away. Nerve pain can also occur after other cancer treatments, such as radiation or chemotherapy.

- *Bone pain*—Cancer can spread into the bone and cause pain. The cancer may affect one specific area of bone or several areas. The cancer cells within the bone damage the bone tissue and cause the pain. People often describe this type of pain as aching, dull, or throbbing.
- *Soft tissue pain*—pain from a body organ or muscle. For example, you may have pain in your back caused by tissue damage to the kidney. You can't always pinpoint this pain, but it is usually described as sharp, cramping, aching, or throbbing. Soft tissue pain is also called visceral pain.
- *Phantom pain*—pain in a part of the body that has been removed. For example, pain in an arm or leg that has been amputated due to sarcoma or osteosarcoma. Or pain in the breast area after mastectomy. Phantom pain is very real, and people sometimes describe it as unbearable.

   Between 60 and 70 percent of people who have had an arm or leg removed feel phantom pain. About one-third of women who have had a breast removed feel phantom breast pain. The pain usually lessens after the first year, but some people can still feel phantom pain after a year or more. In most people it will go away after a few months. It is as though your brain has to realize that part of your body is gone.
- *Referred pain*—pain from an organ in the body that is felt in a different part of the body. For example, a swollen liver may cause pain in the right shoulder, even though the liver is under the ribs on the right side of the body. This is because the liver presses on nerves that pass through the shoulder.

Physical Health Recommendations

The following recommendations will help reduce cancer pain by enhancing cancer management.

Diet

For cancer pain, refer to the anti-inflammatory diet in Chapter 5. Combine this diet with a macrobiotic diet, which is recommended for treating cancer. Analysis of case studies indicates that a strict macrobiotic diet, an extension of a vegetarian diet, is likely to be more effective in long-term cancer management than diets offering a variety of other foods.

Raw fruit and vegetable juices are widely recommended as part of supportive treatment for cancer; they are an easy way to take in over 95 percent of the vital phytonutrients that support the immune system. Organic fruits and vegetables are much preferred.

Vitamins, Minerals, and Supplements

Although their primary focus is not on relieving cancer pain, the following vitamins, minerals, and supplements provide a wide range of support for cancer patients. And if the cancer itself improves, so too does the pain.

In addition to these, there are other products that provide a range of support for cancer patients, including:

- *Antioxidants* exert anti-carcinogenic, immune-stimulant, and anti-metastatic effects and act to inhibit cancer at each stage of its development. Since it is known that platelet aggregation, a free radical–mediated function, encourages implantation of bloodstream-borne cancer metastases, increasing antioxidant intake becomes important. Reasonable daily doses of antioxidants in treating cancer are: selenium, 500 mcg; vitamin E, 800 IU; and vitamin C, 4 gm. Beta carotene (125,000 IU daily) regresses oral (mouth) precancerous lesions. Studies have confirmed the benefits of high-dose antioxidants during chemo- and radiation therapy in both reducing toxicity of treatment and enhancing treatment effects.
- *Lycopene*: a carotenoid that substantially inhibits the growth of lung cancer cells in the test tube and has been shown to reduce progression of prostate cancer (with a dosage of 15 mg daily). Lycopene, a major tomato carotenoid, is ten times more potent than beta-carotene.
- *IV vitamin C*: Linus Pauling and Ewan Cameron reported benefits of intravenous vitamin C in "terminal" cancer patients in 1971. Administered intravenously in high dosages (60–100 gm over ten hours), vitamin C can induce cytotoxicity in tumor cells with negligible toxic effects to normal cells.

- *Probiotics*: The toxicity of chemotherapy routinely disrupts intestinal bacterial balance; restoring acidophilus and bifidus organisms in the intestine promotes normal intestinal function during treatment.

Herbs

- *Genistein*: an isoflavone from fruits and vegetables that, as well as other flavonoids—flavone, luteolin, and daidzein—has been shown to inhibit the growth of stomach cancer cells in test tube experiments. Human squamous skin cancer cells in test tube experiments were significantly inhibited by various concentrations of quercetin (a common flavonoid found in onions, apples, and berries). Reasonable doses for these flavonoids are 400 mg twice daily. Tangeretin, a naturally occurring flavone in citrus fruit, causes cancer cell death in promyelocytic leukemia cells in the test tube. Therefore, large amounts of citrus fruits are encouraged.
- *Maitake mushroom extracts*: have immune-enhancing and anti-cancer properties, and are now being used in the U.S. The recommended dosage is 3 capsules three times daily.
- *Silymarin (Milk Thistle)*: 80 percent standardized extracts are helpful in preserving liver function during chemotherapy treatment with 5-fluorouracil and other agents. The recommended dosage is 140–210 mg two to three times daily.

Biomolecular Options

Anticoagulants reduce the rate of metastases in cancer patients. Some reports have cataloged great reductions in patients who were coincidentally anticoagulated for other reasons. This report has not led to widespread utilization of this observation.

The ability to synthesize the adrenal hormone *dehydroepiandrosterone (DHEA)* declines markedly over the third through sixth decades of life. The levels of DHEA in patients with a wide variety of cancers are found to be generally low. DHEA has been used with benefit as a treatment in some types of cancer.

Glutathione, an antioxidant synthesized by the body, added intravenously to chemotherapeutic cisplatin regimens for advanced ovarian cancer decreased toxicity and significantly improved prognosis.

There is some preliminary evidence that *melatonin* may be helpful in the treatment of cancer. Patients with brain metastases from solid cancers who received melatonin (20 mg daily) in addition to supportive care tripled their aggregate survival time in one year of treatment. Clear improvement in quality of life and performance status was present in 30 percent of the melatonin patients compared to none in the controls. Melatonin (10 mg daily) prevented metastases in 40 percent of patients with far-advanced cancers.

Coenzyme Q10 (100 mg daily) added to cancer treatment prevented the heart toxicity usually developing with Adriamycin (doxorubicin) chemotherapy. Women with breast cancer, advanced liver, and metastatic disease have successfully been treated with 400 mg daily.

Exercise

Physical activity appears to be helpful in the treatment of cancer. In human studies, increased physical activity in cancer patients increases appetite, conserves lean tissue, improves functional capacity, slows the clinical course of the cancer, pushes back the time of death, and improves the quality of life.

More Self-Care Therapies

Several thousand case histories of documented "spontaneous" recovery from cancer have been summarized by Brendan O'Regan and Caryle Hirshberg of the Institute of Noetic Sciences. In many case histories, the "fighting spirit," will to live, and belief in recovery appear to be very important prognostic factors. Most patients who recover from life-threatening cancer have made a radical change in some aspect of their lives—in diet, exercise, attitude, relationships with family members, or sense of connection with God. Other characteristics frequently observed to be present in persons who cure their cancers include full acceptance of their disease and using the occasion of the disease as an opportunity to gain some sense of meaning and purpose in their lives. This introspective journey of self-discovery is often so important to them that many actually feel gratitude for the "gift" of cancer.

Confidence and belief in the program of cancer treatment undertaken seems to be essential in successfully treating cancer. Self-confidence and confidence in the treating physicians are also essential elements. It is very important for patients to participate in decisions regarding their own treatment.

Professional Care Therapies

- *Relaxation training* (9 hours): This has been shown to significantly reduce cancer pain and use of narcotics and tranquilizers. Hypnosis also greatly enhances the management of pain in cancer.
- *Support groups:* Patients with malignant melanoma who were enrolled in an intervention group did better than those in a "routine care" group. The intervention group met one and a half hours weekly for six weeks. Group processes and interventions included health education, cancer education, enhancement of illness-related problem-solving skills, instruction and practice in relaxation skills, psychological support, and promoting interaction between patients and health care professionals. Psychological and immunological testing at six months compared to baseline showed significant improvement in immunity compared to controls, and anxiety and depression were significantly less as well. Imagery enhanced the effects of relaxation on immunity. In a six-year follow-up, the risk of dying was 33 percent less and the risk of recurrence 50 percent less in the intervention group.

   In a landmark study of late-stage female breast cancer patients, a one-year weekly support group including relaxation training greatly enhanced quality of life and more than doubled the survival time of these women. Patients with a solid support system of relatives, spouses, and significant others have a better prognosis, as do married men and men with a confidant.
- *Energy medicine:* In well-controlled animal studies, cancer progression has been shown to be inhibited with energy treatments by healers using therapeutic or Healing Touch, Reiki, or similar hands-on techniques.
- *Mental imagery:* In many of the reports of people recovering from cancer, especially advanced cancer, patients have used imagery of their immune systems overcoming or defeating the cancer cells and imagery

of themselves returning to health. Authoritative research confirms that the success of imagery is highly related to the vividness and effectiveness visualized in the imagery. Guided imagery therapy with skilled professionals in this area can be very helpful and meaningful.

The Issues in Your Tissues

Studies show increases in cancer in people under chronic, excessive, unmanaged stress and especially after acutely stressful events, such as the death of a spouse or other significant losses, including loss of a job or career setbacks. A common denominator in this data is the loss of love, either from oneself or from a significant other. In several studies, the way people cope with stress has been correlated with cancer-related deaths and rate of cancer progression. I have previously made the point that stress/anxiety is a major factor for increasing pain, whether it's cancer pain, nerve pain, or from any other source.

Depression is often associated with cancer incidence. A large number of studies have noticed the consistent significant relationship between depression, helplessness, and hopelessness and the onset of various kinds of cancer. Depressed patients have a much lower incidence of successful bone-marrow-transplant survival than non-depressed patients. Patients who express their emotions in socially acceptable ways rather than repressing them also consistently do better. Behavioral and cognitive therapy can be of enormous help in treating depression.

Medical intuitives and esoteric diagnosticians who are aware of energy fields also sense cancer as a disorder related to negative emotions of fear, guilt, self-hate/self-denial (loss of love from self); unfinished business with others with whom one has had a significant relationship (perceived loss of love from others); and resistance to change (an inability to let go of the past and feel the loss).

These issues create a major impediment to the evolution of emotional, psychological, and spiritual development. Accepting the fact that we experience change according to what our growth requires necessitates the development of a willingness to accept ourselves as we are, to let go of those issues over which we have no control, and to recognize the necessity and inevitability of change in order to grow and incorporate what we need to learn in this lifetime.

Dr. Caroline Bedell Thomas's long-term study of fifteen hundred medical students showed that the strongest psychological predictor of cancer over the next twenty-five years was the perception of a lack of closeness with parents in childhood.

Patient Story—**Cancer Pain**

Ally F. is a twenty-nine-year-old co-owner of a medical marijuana dispensary, who was in excellent health until she was diagnosed with an aggressive form of thyroid cancer at age twenty-five. By the time it was diagnosed, it had already spread to the lymph nodes in her neck. Her treatment included a total thyroidectomy (surgical removal of the entire thyroid gland) in addition to radiation.

Her surgery was successful, with thirty-nine cancerous lymph nodes removed from her neck and upper arm, along with her thyroid. She was given an opioid for pain relief immediately following surgery, but she was not able to tolerate it (nausea and vomiting). Her doctors weren't sure how to treat her, but since she had previously used cannabis for migraines she decided to use it for her postoperative pain.

She used indica edibles, both lozenges and lollipops, to soothe her sore throat and to help with the severe neck pain resulting from the surgery. She felt immediate relief. Several days after the surgery she started radiation. The doctors prescribed a variety of medications, including tramadol, Oxycontin, and hydrocodone, but none of them helped to relieve the pain from the radiation treatments, and each of them caused a similar reaction to the first opioid following surgery—i.e., nausea and vomiting. Once again she obtained significant relief with cannabis.

During the course of the radiation treatment, she spent countless hours vomiting and couldn't eat or sleep: "Only cannabis provided me with both the mental and physical relief to allow me to eat and sleep. One inhale of an indica cannabis strain would allow me to fall asleep. One small candy would stop my nausea, and the topical ointment I used immediately helped with the physical pain immensely.

"After a few days the C-4 nerve in my neck went numb. Something had happened during the surgery and my nerve wasn't talking to my brain anymore. I couldn't use my upper arm. I couldn't lift anything and it was like lightning bolts were running down my arm. I was scared, weak, depressed, and in constant pain. Cannabis helped immediately. I would smoke a few times a day whenever the pain got debilitating. The mental relief was unmatched, and the pain pills I tried made me feel nauseous and sick. I used topical ointments, edibles, and ingestible options to treat the pain, depending on whether I was trying to work and function or get a good night of sleep. I could not fall asleep without smoking or ingesting cannabis in some way. Ultimately cannabis saved my life and provided me with the relief I needed to fight the cancer and win. It helped me both mentally and physically and allowed me to keep working and functioning, and it has become a staple in my life as I deal with the chronic pain still in my arm on a daily basis.

"Luckily I had access to cannabis and was able to use specific strains that were high in cannabidiol (CBD) and not tetrahydrocannabinol (THC). I used these cannabinoids proportionally to the functionality I needed and I learned about treatment in varying degrees. Today I help patients all across Colorado with their chronic pain treatment plans and try to find the best options for each individual. I am confident that cannabis can help chronic pain patients just like it helped me, and I am excited to see the scientific developments rooted around the cannabis plant. I am hopeful that one day people with cancer and other illnesses can use cannabis as an herbal treatment instead of having to suffer through dangerous unnecessary surgery and radiation treatments."

Chapter 15

Emotional Pain: Anxiety, Insomnia, and Depression

I Am Safe, I Am at Peace with Life

ANXIETY

Anxiety is a state of fear or worry in the face of a perceived threat of danger. It is an emotional dis-ease or uneasiness, in which the anxious individual describes feeling tense, nervous, or disturbed. Within the medical community this condition of fear is known as anxiety neurosis, and it affects twice as many women as men. Someone with anxiety manifesting as IBS might feel worried sick, with their "stomach in knots." *Nearly all people with chronic pain also have anxiety.*

There is probably no one who has not experienced at least some degree of anxiety. Like depression (see below), it covers a spectrum of emotional discomfort that ranges from mild appropriate concern to being overwhelmed by an excessive continuous state of worry. In fact, anxiety often accompanies depression, as well as obsessive compulsive disorders and posttraumatic stress disorder (PTSD). When taken to the extreme, anxiety manifests as acute panic attacks and phobias. Generalized anxiety disorder is characterized by *excessive* or unwarranted *worry* (usually over work, finances, relationships, and health) that occurs chronically for at least six months. The degree of fear is often unrelated to any obvious cause. But in today's world, global and financial instability, terrorism, governmental dysfunction, and the divisiveness that presently permeates our society have provided an abundance of obvious contributors to our current epidemic of anxiety and its offspring, insomnia.

Anxiety and fear trigger the "fight-or-flight" response, which causes excess adrenaline to be produced by the adrenal glands along with other hormones called catecholamines, and the body prepares itself for action. When no action is taken and nervous energy is not discharged, there is physiological confusion. This could be described as an anxiety or panic attack, manifested by many of the *symptoms* in the following list:

- Restlessness, irritability, feeling keyed up or on edge/a sense of urgency
- Insomnia (difficulty falling or staying asleep, nightmares)
- Heart palpitations (rapid or irregular heartbeat)
- Muscle tension, especially in the neck, shoulders, and chest
- Easily fatigued
- Difficulty concentrating or mind going blank
- Rapid and shallow breathing, or feeling short of breath (hyperventilation)
- Trembling or feeling shaky
- Dry mouth
- Generalized sweating, or sweaty palms
- Headaches
- Abdominal pain and/or diarrhea
- Loss of appetite
- Occasional panic attacks

Conventional medical treatment for anxiety consists primarily of antianxiety medications, called *benzodiazepines*. These include Xanax (alprazolam), Klonopin (clonazepam), Ativan (lorazepam), and Valium (diazepam). Although these drugs act rapidly and effectively and relieve panic attacks and general anxiety, they can be addictive, impair memory, and increase fatigue. Similar to opioids for treating physical pain, these medications can be quite helpful when used for a short time. Daily, long-term use, however, can be a problem, especially with addiction and deaths from overdose. According to the Centers for Disease Control and Prevention, benzodiazepines were involved in about 30 percent of prescription drug *overdose deaths* in 2013, second only to opioids, which were involved in 70 percent.

MEDICAL MARIJUANA RECOMMENDATIONS FOR ANXIETY

Among my patient population, relief from anxiety is the third-most sought therapeutic benefit from MMJ, behind pain and insomnia. But unlike the top two symptoms, I advise patients suffering with anxiety to avoid significant amounts of THC, unless their anxiety is accompanied by physical pain, which is often the case. This poses somewhat of a challenge to find an effective balance, which must be determined by each individual.

The problem is that anxiety, pain, and insomnia are closely connected. With increased anxiety, your pain is likely to be worse, which can then result in greater difficulty obtaining a good night's sleep. And those who are sleep-deprived are invariably more anxious. This is a miserable cycle, one that I briefly experienced during the height of my bout with shingles, until I discovered the right combination of MMJ products.

As I've previously mentioned, some THC is needed for optimal pain relief, but in someone who has a predisposition toward higher levels of anxiety, too much THC can increase it. What is too much? Individuals must determine that for themselves. A minimal amount of THC—for example, the strongest indica strains (80:20/I:S)—are invariably helpful before bed for inducing sleep and decreasing anxiety. However, many patients with high anxiety also use these same strong indica strains or a 70:30/I:S during the day without feeling the least bit sleepy. In fact they function quite well, and often describe the effect as "it levels me out, and helps me feel more grounded."

Depending on one's level of anxiety, *vaporizing the indica-dominant strains*, 80:20, 70:30, or 60:40, is recommended for patients with *anxiety accompanied by some degree of physical pain*. Indica *edibles*, Stratos Sleep (indica) *tablets*, or Med-a-mints indica *sublingual tablets* are other indica options that work well for both anxiety and sleep, depending on the time of day they are taken. But as with the majority of MMJ products, you'll have to experiment and see what works best for you.

For those patients with *anxiety and no pain*, the high-CBD tinctures with little or no THC are preferred over indica-THC products. Examples of high-CBD tinctures include Charlotte's Web or Restorative Botanicals, both of which are derived from hemp oil.

Other high-CBD products derived from marijuana include 20:1/ CBD:THC tincture, or vaporizing a high-CBD strain of marijuana flower. Also effective are the Stratos tablets, 15:1/CBD:THC; CBD capsules, 25 or 50 mg; or high-CBD edibles.

As a rule with high-CBD products, the lower the percentage of THC, the less effective the product is as an analgesic. However, it will still retain its anxiety-lowering effect. The CBD products derived from hemp oil with less than 1 percent THC are legal and they are the preferred choice for those who do not want to feel even the slightest psychoactive effect. Studies have shown that they are most effective for relieving anxiety, rather than reducing pain or helping with sleep. It is important to note that many people find that a mild psychoactive effect is often helpful in relieving anxiety.

HOLISTIC MEDICAL TREATMENT AND PREVENTION PROGRAM FOR ANXIETY

Risk Factors and Causes

The causes of *anxiety* include:

- Fear—relationships and situations that contribute to insecurity
- Chronic pain or prolonged illness/inflammation
- Excess caffeine
- Excess sugar, chocolate, NutraSweet
- Excess of highly acidic foods—tomatoes, eggplants, peppers
- Stimulants—decongestants, NoDoz, tobacco, and asthma and corticosteroid medications
- Hyperthyroidism
- Hyperadrenalism
- Hypoglycemia
- Nutritional deficiencies of B vitamins and magnesium

- History of trauma: physical, sexual, or emotional abuse
- Abnormal levels of stress hormones and/or neurotransmitters

Physical Health Recommendations

Functional Medicine Testing

Holistic and Functional Medicine practitioners can now accurately measure your chemistry of stress:

> Levels of *neurotransmitters*, such as serotonin, GABA, dopamine, glutamate, norepinephrine, epinephrine, and PEA, can be measured with a simple urine test. If it is determined that you have an abnormal level, there are support therapies that can either help to reduce excess stimulatory neurotransmitters that might be causing or aggravating anxiety, or boost relaxation chemicals like serotonin and GABA. With this testing your practitioner can help to personalize your holistic treatment program. For the past decade this approach has proven to be highly successful for significantly reducing or eliminating anxiety. The neurotransmitter test can be performed by NeuroScience Pharmasan Labs.

> The adrenal stress hormones cortisol and DHEA can be measured with a saliva test. These stress hormones are associated with the body's "fight-or-flight" system. Many people with anxiety and/or sleep disorders have elevated cortisol, which is stimulating, and depressed or elevated DHEA. Labs performing this test include Genova, NeuroScience Pharmasan Labs, and Diagnos-Techs, among others (see Resources for URLs).

Diet

The recommended diet for treating anxiety includes complex carbohydrates (whole grains—especially brown rice, barley, millet, non-GMO corn, and original wheat [that has not been hybridized]), vegetables, seaweed, and foods containing L-tryptophan (sunflower seeds, bananas, milk [unless you are dairy sensitive]). These foods support serotonin production. The diet is moderate in protein, fat (30 percent of calories), and strong spices. Caffeine, chocolate, alcohol, sugar, and highly acidic foods should be avoided.

Vitamins, Minerals, and Supplements

- *Gamma-amino butyric acid (GABA)*: a nonessential amino acid in the brain that the body uses to calm anxiety naturally. Most tranquilizers (Xanax, Ativan, Valium, etc.) create a calming effect by stimulating the natural GABA receptors. But unlike tranquilizers, the common oral form of GABA from the health food store cannot pass the blood-brain barrier and is believed to be ineffective in calming the brain. However, it is very helpful in relieving anxiety symptoms originating in the digestive tract and adjacent organs—for example, diarrhea, "stomach butterflies," heart palpitations, and hyperventilation. This is due to its effect on what some scientists refer to as the second, or GI, brain (see Chapter 10). It may take several weeks to appreciate the full benefit of GABA. There is a form of it called pharmaGABA that is well absorbed and readily available in most health food stores. The recommended dosage for daytime relaxation is up to 750 mg two times daily. For *sleep*, take 500–1,500 mg before bed. There is a form of GABA called Phenibut that does cross the blood-brain barrier, and is contained in some NeuroScience products.

- *RelaxMax* (Xymogen): a tasty powder containing L-theanine, an amino acid that helps potentiate GABA in the nervous system. Theanine will begin having an effect within twenty minutes. It also contains myo-inositol, a supplement well documented to reduce anxiety, as well as super-absorbable magnesium and taurine. The recommended dosage is 1–2 scoops one to three times daily in cool water between meals.

- *5-HTP or 5-hydroxytryptophan* is often quite effective for dealing with anxiety. This amino acid is readily converted into *serotonin*, which is a calming neurotransmitter as well as an antidepressant. It is best taken on an empty stomach for absorption and conversion. The recommended dosage for anxiety of 100–200 mg twice a day between meals is often sufficient. As a *sleep* aid, take 50–200 mg before bedtime. I recommend Xymogen's 5-HTP CR. It is time-released and works slowly and steadily.

- *Vitamin C*: Take at least 1,000 mg three times daily.

- *Vitamin B complex or B Activ* (Xymogen): Take 1 capsule at breakfast and lunch daily. This is a scientifically formulated B complex with methylated B vitamins that are essential for the production of anti-stress neurotransmitters, and for balancing adrenal hormones.

    NOTE: A very small percentage of people will have increased anxiety with vitamin B complex.
- *Essential fatty acids (EFAs)/OmegaGenics EPA/DHA 720* (Metagenics): a high-dose, pharmaceutical-grade fish oil. (Fish oil has been shown to lower anxiety.) The recommended dosage is 1–3 capsules daily with meals.

Herbs

- *Kava kava (Piper methysticum)*: an herb that has been successfully used by herbalists since the discovery of its use in Polynesia by Captain James Cook. It is used for treating anxiety and promoting *sleep*. Kava kava is one of the best-studied herbs with proven effectiveness, as well as being one of the best known and utilized. Kava kava is available in both liquid and capsule form. Use the standardized extract of its active ingredient, kavalactone. For daytime relief of anxiety, take 250 mg (one capsule or one-half dropperful) three times daily with meals. One can take four to six capsules for *sleep* (up to 1,500 mg). As with all other medications and nutrients, each individual has a biochemical individuality and needs to take responsibility for finding his or her own unique level. Kava kava should not be taken continuously for a prolonged period of time (more than four months).
- *Valerian*: the treatment of choice for over two hundred years throughout the world for anxiety and *insomnia*. Although it is quite safe to take for short periods of time, its long-term effects are not known. For daytime anxiety, the recommended dosage is 150 mg (standardized extract of 0.8 percent valeric acid) three times daily. For difficulty with *sleep*, start with 150 mg, forty-five minutes before bed. If that dose is insufficient, gradually increase to 600 mg.
- Other herbs that can be used for treating anxiety include chamomile, passionflower, lemon balm, and skullcap. The latter two are best for acute anxiety.

If the above herbs are not helping, there are stronger herbal formulas that holistic practitioners can recommend.

Exercise

Longer, low-intensity aerobic exercise requiring greater endurance, such as jogging, swimming, and hiking, is best for relieving anxiety. Tai chi, yoga, and qigong are also excellent.

Professional Care Therapies

The following therapies can all be effective in treating anxiety: acupuncture (especially five-element style) and traditional Chinese medicine (TCM), Ayurvedic medicine, biofeedback training, bodywork (especially Rolfing), breathwork, chiropractic, environmental medicine (including detoxification therapy), homeopathy, mind-body medicine (guided imagery, meditation, hypnotherapy, neurolinguistic programming), naturopathic medicine, psychotherapy, and professional counseling (especially cognitive therapy).

Stress-Reduction Techniques

Each of the following can be helpful in treating both *anxiety* and *depression*:

- *Meditation*: a technique for calming the mind. A sound or mantra can be used as an "object of meditation." Transcendental meditation uses a repetitive phrase to focus one's attention. Another method is to focus attention on the breath or other body sensations, a technique used in Vipassana and Zen meditation. Raja yoga is an integrative transpersonal approach that elicits responses of intuition and creativity. Whatever the specific method, the goal is to build confidence, increase focus and concentration, and reduce anxiety and depression. Thus, the feedback loop—consisting of depressive thinking, anxiety, hopeless feelings, more depressive thinking—is diminished.
- *Relaxation training*: teaches you to relax the body by progressively tensing and relaxing various muscle groups. Variations include tensing your fists while rolling your eyes upward and holding your breath. You then sequentially relax the eyes, exhale, and release the tension in your

fists. This produces a "letting go" effect that can then be enhanced by focusing on counting down from five to one, picturing each number in a different color. Unlike meditation, this method emphasizes physical relaxation. Since you can't think depressing thoughts while physically relaxing, this method is effective for relaxing the mind as well.

- *Breath techniques*: include several breathing methods derived from yoga and various forms of meditation. More recently, these practices have been used with good effect by patients of psychotherapy to calm the mind and body. Sometimes called *breath therapy*, the techniques include quickly paced, connected (no pause between inhalation and exhalation) mouth breathing (to evoke emotions). Breath therapy allows repressed emotions to surface and be released. Alternating mouth-nose breathing is good for centering, and alternating nostril breathing can enhance creativity. Some of these breathing techniques can be enhanced with imagery and music. Each breathing method has its own intention and rationale and can be quite helpful in treating anxiety and depression. To get started, work with a qualified breath therapist. These methods are quite easy to learn and highly effective.

- *Biofeedback training*: a systematized approach for learning relaxation that provides feedback evidence of reaching a calmer level of brain-wave activity and physiological response. By allowing you to refocus energy in a self-empowering way, it gives you a greater feeling of control over your autonomic ("involuntary") nervous system reactions (heart rate, blood pressure), including those triggered by stress. With the help of a biofeedback technician, you are hooked up to an apparatus that measures your responses (heart rate, muscle tension, skin temperature, brain waves) while you focus on a sensory cue to help you relax. If you need technical confirmation that something is happening, this method is for you. During the past decade, *breath feedback* using capnometry (measures CO_2) has been highly effective in helping to relieve anxiety, pain, and depression.

- *Journaling*: a technique for recording your emotions and understanding patterns of action based on your feelings. To begin to focus on positive experiences, try keeping a *gratitude journal*. This consists of writing each day about something for which you can be grateful. By making a gratitude entry each evening before bed, you neutralize the mind-set that focuses on what's wrong in your life—the depression cycle—and you begin to appreciate what's right.

- *Hypnosis (hypnotherapy)*: a form of treatment that can be quite effective with milder types of anxiety and depression. Hypnosis produces an *altered state of consciousness* (ASC) in which certain senses are heightened and others seem to fade into the background. It is not a state of sleep. While in a hypnotic trance, you become more aware of words and suggested images, and they grow more intense.

    Bodily sensations and time are often distorted. You do not need a deep trance to receive the benefits of hypnosis; a light trance is often adequate. Images of calm, relaxing scenes are often suggested for clients with anxiety. Although the visual imagery is quite effective, much of the benefit from hypnosis is obtained by the simple act of learning to relax. It is often a revelation to learn that you *can* relax.

    Depression is often a pattern of seeing yourself and your life with a bleak sense of entrapment. Hypnotherapy can be used to imagine, while in a heightened state of suggestibility, more hopeful options and better methods of dealing with painful issues. While in a hypnotic state, one can visually rehearse newer ways of perceiving oneself.

- *Self-hypnosis*: which can easily be learned from a skilled therapist (and even from books), provides simple and effective methods for training yourself to enter a hypnotic state. Audiotapes are also an excellent source of training in self-hypnosis and learning strategies to relax and reprogram habits of the mind.

- *Emotional Freedom Techniques (EFT)*: an energy psychology technique that can be quite helpful in treating anxiety, depression, and insomnia. Utilizing acupressure, EFT's central premise is that the cause of all painful emotions is a disruption in the body's energy system. Although it can be an effective self-care technique with practice, it is best to learn it from a trained practitioner. Also known as "Tapping," there are several websites (e.g., thetappingsolution.com) with a wealth of information on EFT.

- *Progressive muscle relaxation*: another form of hypnotherapy that is effective for anxiety. The client is instructed to start by tensing, then relaxing, the muscles of the feet, then repeating this process with each muscle group in succession, moving all the way up the body to the face and forehead (similar to relaxation training, described above).

- *Self-talk*: re-scripting self-dialogue from self-defeating to positive encouragement. This is done through the use of affirmations or changing phrases from "if only" to "I am!"
- *NLP* (neuro-linguistic programming): has proven extremely successful with intractable phobias and certain forms of anxiety. It utilizes transformational imagery to modify behavior and help reshape emotional patterns.
- Spending consistent time immersed in *creative activities* such as painting or playing a musical instrument can help with anxiety and depression. The same holds true for daily and weekly scheduled time for *play and/or relaxation*, as well as periodic *vacations*.

The Issues in Your Tissues

The mental and emotional health techniques most effective for anxiety include psychotherapy; stress-reduction techniques—meditation, relaxation training, breath therapy, and biofeedback training; journaling; energy medicine—Healing and Therapeutic Touch, Reiki, qigong, along with working on the specific emotional issues associated with your condition; hypnosis; bodywork therapies; planned retreats and vacations—even long weekends away from home are helpful; creative activities—art, music.

Spiritual Health Recommendations

Holistic medicine is based on the belief that unconditional love is life's most powerful healer. Love and fear are inversely proportional—i.e., the greater one's capacity for love, the less one's fear. *Spiritual psychotherapy* is focused on expanding one's capacity for self-love. Since fear is the primary cause of anxiety, those spiritual practices that are most beneficial for reducing fear are also the most helpful for lessening anxiety. These include prayer, psalms (especially Psalms 23 [before bed], 91 [after work], and 121 [early morning, facing east), meditation, and altruism (volunteering).

Patient Story—**Anxiety**

Richard U. is a sixty-three-year-old trial attorney who, since his divorce twelve years ago, had been taking Ativan (2 mg) two to three times daily to relieve his anxiety. He also had moderate pain in both knees from osteoarthritis.

He began using MMJ approximately one year ago, and although his job is no less stressful and he's not been in counseling as I had recommended, he's been able to wean himself off the Ativan and now uses it no more than once or twice a week. He typically vaporizes the stronger indica strains of MMJ (some with high-CBD content), either 70:30 or 80:20/I:S, and functions quite well during the day, without the least bit of drowsiness. According to Richard, "it levels me out." In the evening or after work, he tends to do the heaviest indica strains, which he says help him to relax.

He will also occasionally use indica edibles early in the day. He finds that he's able to obtain some relief from his arthritic pain with the indica flower and edibles, in addition to the topical cream Apothecanna Extra Strength.

Richard's case of anxiety is somewhat unusual in that it did not respond at all to CBD tincture (with no THC), or any of the anti-anxiety supplements that I recommended. This may be indicative of an especially severe case of anxiety, or possibly not being patient long enough to determine the appropriate dose of the CBD tincture or the supplements.

However, he seems satisfied with the results he's obtained from the indica and has been able to nearly stop the Ativan entirely, which was his original objective.

INSOMNIA

Just as the incidence of anxiety has increased dramatically during the past two decades, so too has insomnia. Insomnia is our most common type of sleep disorder, defined as a *lack of sleep due to insufficient quality or quantity* and typically involves *difficulty falling asleep or staying asleep*. Most cases of insomnia are caused by varying degrees of *anxiety*. Insomnia also occurs as a result of medical conditions (especially chronic pain, heart disease, and cancer), depression, medications, and environmental factors (e.g., temperature extremes, noise, light), changes in sleep habits, and lack of exercise.

Sleep apnea is one of the less common but potentially most serious types of secondary insomnia. It is a disorder in which there is intermittent cessation of breathing during sleep, which forces the individual to repeatedly wake up to take breaths. It affects predominantly men between thirty and sixty.

The most common *symptoms* accompanying insomnia are fatigue, immune deficiencies (increased susceptibility to illness), headaches, weight gain, irritability, depression, slowed reaction time, diminished short-term memory, decreased libido, poor job performance, and increased substance abuse.

Why do we need to sleep, and why does sleep have such a profound impact on our physical well-being? Science has been seriously exploring the physiology of sleep since the early 1970s, but it still remains largely a mystery. Although many prominent people (JFK, President Clinton, Martha Stewart, Jay Leno) have claimed they need only three to four hours of sleep, the evidence supports the fact that while sleep requirements are highly individualized, most people require seven to eight hours to function optimally. Even as the quality of sleep diminishes with age, the need for sleep does not.

There are two distinct physiological states of sleep: non–rapid eye movement (NREM—deep sleep), with four stages defined by specific electroencephalogram (EEG) features, and REM sleep, characterized by episodic bursts of rapid eye movements, muscle relaxation, and dream activity. The two types of sleep alternate throughout the night, in three to six ninety-minute NREM-REM cycles.

The functional purposes of NREM and REM sleep states are not definitively known. However, most sleep researchers accept the idea that the purpose of NREM sleep is at least in part restorative—i.e., replenishing immune cells; restoring organs, bones, and tissue; and circulating a rejuvenating supply of growth hormone, making us less vulnerable to the diseases of aging. Studies show that when deprived of sleep, the brain prioritizes deep sleep over REM sleep. Although the function of REM sleep remains a matter of considerable controversy, some studies indicate that it is crucial for proper functioning of the brain and psyche. While more research is needed, it's possible that the ability of marijuana to increase deep sleep, even at the expense of REM sleep, might turn out to be a good thing.

MEDICAL MARIJUANA RECOMMENDATIONS FOR INSOMNIA

Numerous studies have shown that using marijuana before bed *reduces REM sleep and lengthens the time the brain spends in deep sleep (NREM)*. Most of these studies on marijuana and sleep have looked primarily at the effects of THC, and do not reflect the predominance of strong indicas (with relatively small amounts of THC) currently used by the vast majority of MMJ patients for sleep. I continue to hear repeatedly from my patients that the greatest benefit they derive from MMJ is better quality sleep, with pain relief and decreased anxiety a close second and third. As I've explained in the "Anxiety" section above, these three symptoms are very closely connected.

Researchers believe that marijuana users report fewer dreams because THC reduces REM sleep. Using THC or marijuana before bed also appears to reduce the density of rapid eye movements during REM sleep. Interestingly, less REM density has been linked to more restful sleep.

Although the science of marijuana and its effect on sleep remains unclear, there is nothing ambiguous about the clinical reports I receive from patients on a daily basis as to its tremendous benefits for sleep. And in the majority of cases, marijuana, as indica, has allowed them to stop using their prescription sleep medications.

Remember that all indica strains have some THC, and even though they are an excellent choice for promoting sleep as well as reducing pain, it's easy to take too high a dose. This is especially true with edibles and tinctures, which is why it's best to start out with a minimal dose and gradually increase. Otherwise you might get too high to fall asleep, and if you take too much of an edible or tincture, you can be up for several hours, precisely the opposite effect that you were hoping for. If this occurs, don't worry. If nothing else, it will only last for a few hours before the effect dissipates, and you will have learned a valuable lesson about dosage.

MEDICAL MARIJUANA RECOMMENDATIONS FOR FALLING ASLEEP

- Vaporizing a strong (80:20/I:S) indica strain a few minutes before getting into bed—every dispensary has several options from which to choose. Purchase smaller amounts (e.g., one-eighth ounce) of three or four strains and rotate these strains every two or three days. If you use the same strain every night, you'll develop a tolerance and the effect will gradually weaken. Start with two or three inhalations from a vaporizer (or one or two hits of smoke) at most.
- High-CBD hash oil in a vaporizer pen works well.
- High-CBD tincture—forty to sixty minutes before going to bed. You'll have to experiment to determine the optimum number of drops or sprays for you. Start with three to five drops or sprays of tincture. Best taken on an empty stomach.
- High-CBD hash oil—ingest a 6:1, 12:1, or 20:1 oil in an amount approximately the size of one grain of rice.
- Tinctures or capsules combining CBN/CBD/THC are very effective, especially Prana P4 Bio Medicinals, but at the present time are not readily available outside of California.
- Indica tablets (Stratos Sleep)—ingest between sixty and ninety minutes before bed, along with a fatty food (increases absorption), such as peanut butter, avocado, nuts, cheese. Start with one-half tablet.
- Sublingual indica tablets (MED-a-mints)—dissolve one under your tongue (try and keep it in your mouth for at least ten minutes after it has dissolved) thirty to fifty minutes before bed. Start with one-half tablet.
- CBN—either Mary's Medicinals CBN capsules, transdermal CBN gel pen, or CBN transdermal patch work extremely well for both sleep and pain.
- Indica edibles—require a period of experimentation to determine the best dose. Ingest sixty to ninety minutes before bed and start with a very small piece, approximately one-quarter to one-half of the recommended dose. If there's no effect within ninety minutes, then eat a little more.
- Dixie Elixirs Bath Soak and Mary Jane's Medicinals Hash Bath are both effective for helping to fall asleep.

MEDICAL MARIJUANA RECOMMENDATIONS FOR STAYING ASLEEP

- The indica edibles (six to eight hours), tinctures (four to six hours), Stratos Sleep tablets (six to eight hours), MED-a-mint sublingual tablets (four to six hours), and especially the CBN patch (ten to twelve hours) might last long enough to help you to both fall asleep and stay asleep. This includes easily falling back to sleep if you awaken to urinate during the night.
- Vaporizing in the middle of the night can be an ideal solution for staying asleep as well as falling asleep. If your problem is only waking too early, but you fall asleep OK, then have your vaporizer loaded with a strong indica and set the correct temperature, which is approximately 375 degrees Fahrenheit (assuming you're able to set the exact temperature, as is the case with a good quality vaporizer). Then turn the vaporizer off and set it on the nightstand or table next to your bed, and it will be ready to use if you need it during the night.
- Another option for "middle of the night use" is the Charlotte's Web Disposable CBD Vape Pen.
- If you vaporized before bed to help fall asleep and you have a problem of awakening too early, then before turning the vaporizer off, set the temperature for 390–395 degrees Fahrenheit and place it on your nightstand. One of the advantages of vaporizers is that you can use the same strain a second time if you raise the temperature fifteen to twenty degrees. Although there's more "smoke"—i.e., visible vapor at the higher temperature—this allows you to avoid turning on lights, grinding, and reloading the vaporizer, and in the process becoming more awake.

What Happens When Quitting

Regular users of cannabis experience an abnormal increase in REM sleep when use is stopped. This is called the REM rebound effect, which leads to longer and denser periods of REM sleep. The REM rebound explains why cannabis users often experience highly vivid dreaming when trying to quit.

The sleep disturbances that occur during cannabis withdrawal usually begin twenty-four to seventy-two hours after quitting and can persist for up to six to seven weeks.

The rebound effect appears to be the body's way of coping with being deprived of certain stages of sleep.

HOLISTIC MEDICAL TREATMENT AND PREVENTION PROGRAM FOR INSOMNIA

Risk Factors and Causes

Physical and Environmental

- Age—sleep quality begins to diminish after age forty.
- Inflammation—If you are chronically inflamed, the inflammation will increase neurotransmitters that are stimulatory, such as glutamate, dopamine, epinephrine, PEA, and norepinephrine. This is part of the "fight-or-flight" mechanism. It can also disrupt sleep by increasing nighttime cortisol released from the adrenal glands.
- Lighted screens too late into the evening, such as computers, tablets, phones, and TVs—the lights can reduce melatonin production and keep cortisol levels high at night.
- Menopause—estrogen deficiency.
- PMS—progesterone insufficiency.
- Excess caffeine—in coffee, tea, soft drinks, chocolate, over-the-counter drugs (analgesics and diet pills).
- Drugs—decongestants, thyroid medications, oral contraceptives, beta blockers, marijuana (especially sativa and high-THC products), and overuse of sleep-inducing drugs.
- Stimulating herbs—ginseng, ephedra/ma huang, ginger, guarana, kola nut.
- Sugar (in some sensitive individuals).
- Nocturnal hypoglycemia.
- Allergies.
- Pain.
- Alcohol—initially sedating but lightens sleep as the night goes on.

- Environmental factors—noise, light, temperature, humidity, uncomfortable mattress.
- Insufficient exercise.
- Hypo- and hyperthyroidism; adrenal hyperactivity.
- Chemical hypersensitivity.

Mental/Emotional

- Anxiety, especially the fear of not sleeping.
- Depression.
- Grief.
- Excitement/mania.
- Anticipation of confrontational situations.
- Work stress.

Social/Spiritual

The underlying societal cause of this critical problem is that we are an overworked and overstimulated culture that is continually under pressure to accomplish more in less time. Insomnia is clearly a dis-ease of our modern age. As technology helps us to achieve our material goals, we are sacrificing our relationships, our health, and our happiness.

Physical and Environmental Health Recommendations

Functional Medicine Testing

A neurotransmitter/adrenal cortisol/melatonin test, *NeuroSLP*, is now available through NeuroScience Pharmasan Labs. It is performed by collecting a urine and saliva sample during the night. With this test your holistic practitioner can determine your exact nighttime sleep chemistry.

Diet

Eliminate or reduce all caffeine in your diet, including coffee, tea, chocolate, and cola soft drinks. Also eliminate any other stimulants, such as cigarettes, over-the-counter drugs containing caffeine, hot spicy foods (especially cayenne), sugar, refined carbohydrates (they deplete B vitamins), alcohol (can lighten sleep), food additives, pork (bacon, ham, sausage), eggplant, spinach, and tomatoes. Some people with insomnia suffer from food sensitivities. The most common offending foods are dairy products, wheat and gluten grains, corn, and chocolate. Eliminate all of these foods for three to four weeks, then gradually reintroduce them, except chocolate. Avoid eating a heavy meal before bed, and establish a regular eating schedule.

Foods that enhance sleep have a high tryptophan-to-tyrosine (or phenylalanine) ratio (such as pumpkins, potatoes, bananas, onions, spinach, broccoli, cauliflower, eggs, fish, liver, milk, peanuts, cheddar cheese, whole grains [especially whole wheat, brown rice, and oats], cottage cheese, and beans). Eating tryptophan-rich foods for the evening meal or an evening snack may help induce sleep, including organic milk products from grass-fed cows, turkey, chicken, beef, soy products, nuts and nut butters, bananas, papayas, and figs. If you are hypoglycemic, follow a diet that stabilizes that condition.

Foods that are high in carbohydrates raise the level of serotonin in the brain, which has a sedating effect. Without overeating, you can try having some bean soup, half a baked sweet or Yukon gold potato, cooked root vegetables, or a piece of toast half an hour before bed. Fruits, especially mulberries and lemons, can calm the mind. Drinking an adequate amount of water during the day will prevent waking up at night thirsty. But avoid drinking large amounts before going to sleep.

Vitamins, Minerals, and Supplements

- *Vitamin B complex or B Activ (Xymogen)*: 1 capsule at breakfast and lunch
- *Calcium and magnesium or Ossapan MD (Xymogen)*: within forty-five minutes of bedtime
- *5-Hydroxytryptophan or 5-HTP CR (Xymogen)*: 100 to 200 mg before bed
- *Phosphatidylserine*: up to 100–300 mg daily with dinner; an amino acid for those with insomnia due to elevated cortisol levels, usually induced by stress
- *GABA*: Either *PharmaGABA*, as mentioned above for anxiety, or a professional type of GABA that passes through the blood-brain barrier. This must be done with holistic medical supervision.

- *Hormones*: *Melatonin* is a normally occurring hormone manufactured and released by the pineal gland in response to darkness. It is most effective for the type of insomnia that manifests primarily as difficulty falling asleep, and its recommended dosage ranges from 1 to 4 mg, a half hour to one hour before bed. Melatonin can also be used for sleep maintenance with a sustained-release 1 mg preparation. There is also benefit with melatonin in treating jet lag. One of the best melatonin products is *Melatonin CR* (Xymogen). It has an initial quick release for falling asleep, then a sustained release after that for staying asleep. Take 1 tablet approximately twenty minutes prior to bedtime.

  Natural *progesterone* has been used with good results for insomnia associated with menopause and PMS. Progesterone restores hormonal balance and has a calming effect. Only try this with holistic medical supervision. The majority of menopausal women need natural estrogen support to maintain healthy sleep.

Herbs

- *Benesom (Metagenics)*: a highly effective sleep aid with the following ingredients: calcium, magnesium, Chinese skullcap, passionflower, *Melissa* lemon balm, valerian, hops, and melatonin. The recommended dosage is 1–2 tablets one hour before sleep. *NOTE:* This product contains melatonin. Only add more melatonin under holistic medical supervision.
- *Kava kava*: useful for both anxiety and insomnia. The recommended dosage for sleep is 2 or 3 capsules (60 to 75 mg per capsule) an hour before bedtime.
- *Chinese herbs (and acupuncture)*: often produce dramatic and long-lasting relief from insomnia, but you'll need to find a qualified Chinese medicine practitioner or OMD (doctor of Oriental medicine).

Exercise

Exercising during the afternoon or early evening, five to six hours before bedtime, and avoiding strenuous exercise in the evening is best. *Outdoor exercise* is preferable, since studies show that people who get adequate natural sunlight tend to sleep better. Exercise for at least twenty to thirty minutes—brisk walking, jogging, bicycling, hiking, swimming, or yoga.

Sunlight

Clinical research shows that about thirty minutes of exposure to bright light within two hours of waking can ameliorate sleep disorders, depression, and seasonal affective disorder. This can be from direct sunlight or from full-spectrum indoor lights.

While it's best to take in light within two hours of waking up, there's good news for those who work nights or just can't stand to get up earlier: the important point is to get light before what is called the *circadian nadir*, which most people experience in the mid- to late afternoon. After that, your body begins its downswing toward sleep, and bright light will just throw things off. It can also be beneficial to take your lunch break outside or hold a midday meeting in the sunniest conference room.

Sunshine (or fake sunshine from full-spectrum lights) triggers a chemical message to the hypothalamus that tells the body it's time to wake up and also shuts down the production of melatonin. In addition, exposure to light stimulates the production of serotonin. So morning sunlight helps you out in two major ways: it makes you feel alert and cheery now, and it promotes sleep later. Start the day with sun, and you'll set the stage for a good night's sleep.

Hydrotherapy

Since sleep comes most easily when body temperature is falling, this process can be triggered by soaking in a *warm bath* or hot tub (below 105 degrees; if too hot, it can be stimulating) an hour to ninety minutes before getting into bed. Try keeping the bedroom temperature moderately cool (low sixties) to enhance the effect. To maximize the relaxation of tense muscles, you can add six to eight drops of *lavender oil* (used by aromatherapists for both anxiety and insomnia) and one cup of *Epsom salt* (consists primarily of magnesium, which relaxes muscles) to the bathwater. For maximum relaxation, a massage with lavender or chamomile oil following the bath is ideal.

Sleep Hygiene

- Make sure your bed is comfortable; most people do well with a medium-firm mattress that has a medium-soft top layer of padding.

- Restrict the bed to sleeping and sexual activity only; use other rooms for TV, reading, or conflict resolution.
- If you cannot fall asleep, or wake up and can't go back to sleep, then get up and go into another room and do something boring, including housework, until you're drowsy enough to go back to bed.
- Avoid taking naps.
- Go to sleep at the same time every night, at least eight hours before you have to get up, and set the alarm for the same time every morning; the best quality sleep can be found between 10 pm and 6 am.
- Create optimum bedroom conditions—avoid bright lights after 9 pm. If it's noisy, buy a white noise generator or use foam earplugs; if it's dry, use a warm mist humidifier.
- Avoid obsessing about sleep, and turn the face of the clock away from you.
- Create a relaxing ritual before bed—read, listen to soothing music, do breathing exercises to quiet your mind.
- Lovemaking before sleep will usually induce good quality deep sleep.

The Issues in Your Tissues

The following mental and emotional health options to help you relax and reduce anxiety are recommended just before bedtime:

- Meditation, with or without a mantra.
- Visualization, with or without audiotapes.
- Relaxing breathing exercises, with or without coordinating affirmations. (For example, repeat along with the breath: "I am sleeping soundly and peacefully.")
- Journaling.
- Attitudinal adjustment to reduce fear of insomnia. (Remember that even a couple of hours of sleep is adequate for basic survival; the less anxiety about insomnia, the better you'll sleep.)
- For night-awakening problems, affirm at bedtime that you will remember the thought of your unconscious mind as you awaken, and provide pen and paper on your bedside table. On awakening during the night, allow yourself to come to sufficiently full wakefulness to turn on the light and record a sentence or two about the first thoughts that come to mind.

They will usually relate to the issue with which your unconscious mind has been struggling and stressing you into wakefulness. Several nights may be required to zero in on the topic. Once identified, the issue can be dealt with. Sleep is often dramatically better after using this technique.

Patient Story—**Insomnia**

Margaret B. is a sixty-five-year-old retired psychotherapist with intermittent neck and upper back pain, but her primary reason for using MMJ is for sleep. It has enabled her to stop the prescription sleep aids that she'd been taking for nearly fifteen years, since the onset of menopause.

She rotates several different marijuana products and has been quite pleased with the results. None of them have caused the unpleasant side effects (e.g., hangover effect) she experienced with both Ambien and Trazadone. She had also used Ativan for a brief period of time.

She recognizes that anxiety is a significant cause of her sleep problems, which can be both falling asleep and, more often, staying asleep. When she awakens to go to the bathroom in the middle of the night, she often has trouble falling back to sleep. She has successfully addressed the problem by using a variety of MMJ products.

She most often uses indica edibles (about an hour before bed), which last for six to eight hours, but during the past year she has also started using Stratos Sleep tablets (six to eight hours' duration) with excellent results. Another option that has worked is to vaporize a strong indica just before bed. Rather than emptying the chamber, she increases the temperature setting by fifteen to twenty degrees before turning the vaporizer off, and then places it on the night table by her bed. If she awakens and can't fall back to sleep, she turns on the vaporizer, and with the same leaves but at a twenty-degree higher temperature, she's able to quickly fall back to sleep.

In recent months she's added the MED-a-mints indica sublingual tablets to her rotation. Since these have a somewhat shorter duration than other products (four to six hours), she takes one-half tablet about a half hour before bed, and then if she awakens too early, she takes the other half.

She describes medical marijuana as a "life-changer": "Having a good night's sleep on a regular basis has made a huge difference in my life. I'm so much happier, and I have more energy and much less anxiety."

DEPRESSION

Depression is an all-inclusive term covering the spectrum from major depression at one extreme, to adjustment problems, sadness, and the blues at the other. In the middle of the spectrum are the bulk of depressed people, with chronic, mild, or intermittent depression. *Nearly all people with chronic pain are also suffering from some degree of chronic depression.*

According to the *DSM-5* (the handbook of the American Psychiatric Association), one needs to display at least five of the following nine symptoms for at least two weeks to be diagnosed with a *major depressive disorder*, and one of these five has to be either depressed mood or loss of interest or pleasure in activities.

- Depressed mood for most of the day
- Markedly diminished interest or pleasure in usual activities
- Insomnia or excessive sleep nearly every day
- Significant loss of weight or appetite when not dieting or weight gain
- Agitated or markedly slowed movements nearly every day
- Loss of energy or fatigue nearly every day
- Feelings of worthlessness or inappropriate guilt
- Diminished ability to think or concentrate, or indecisiveness nearly every day
- Recurrent thoughts of death (not just fear of dying), recurrent suicidal thoughts with or without a specific plan

Typically, if you're depressed you have a significant loss of self-esteem, motivation, energy, sense of purpose, and sexual drive. Other typical symptoms include crying spells, self-loathing, irritability and short temper, extreme pessimism, and thoughts of death. Everything seems hopelessly futile.

When the symptoms of the milder and more common forms of depression (the blues) increase in frequency, intensity, and duration, they can become more disabling. Sufferers' relationships, work, and general functioning become more impaired. At that point, when one's symptoms and functioning are clearly perceived as distressing, one has a major depression, and treatment is required. At least 40 percent of people with depression are neither medically diagnosed nor undergo professional treatment, and are therefore not included in the official estimates of the incidence of depression in the United States.

Depression in its various forms currently afflicts about 25 million people in the United States (those who have been diagnosed and are being treated), but the actual number is estimated to be somewhere between 40 and 50 million. This disorder does not distinguish among age, race, culture, or occupation—it is pervasive in all echelons of society. More than twice as many women are being treated for depression than men, but it is not known whether this is because women are more likely to be depressed or because men tend to deny their depression. Suicide rates, especially for younger people, continue to rise. Some studies of high school students reveal that as many as 30 percent commonly think of suicide and feel hopeless. Depressed people are much more likely to develop cancer, die from a second heart attack, or die prematurely. The estimated yearly cost to this country of depression is $50 billion. According to the World Health Organization (WHO), depression is currently the fourth leading cause of disability in the world. Major depressions occur in the course of a lifetime for 10 to 20 percent of the world's population. By the year 2020, WHO estimates that depression will be second only to heart disease as the world's leading chronic disease.

Conventional treatment for depression consists of medication and psychotherapy. Although none of the antidepressant medications are addicting, they can become a psychological crutch, and there is also some evidence that they may speed the recurrence of depression. Multiple studies have also shown that for mild to moderate depression, treatment with antidepressant medication is no better than a placebo. In other words, *the medication may have little or no therapeutic benefit.*

The combination of medication and conventional psychotherapy alone, without treatment of the body and spirit, is often not effective for treating moderate to severe depression.

MEDICAL MARIJUANA RECOMMENDATIONS FOR DEPRESSION

The majority of patients suffering with depression favor sativa strains of MMJ, since the THC improves mood, increases energy and appetite, and enhances their ability to focus on whatever activity they are engaged in. For those whose depression is accompanied by some degree of anxiety, which includes a large segment of the depressed population, hybrids are the preferred choice. They can be either 50:50 or 60:40/S:I. These should be vaporized (vape pen hybrid hash oil cartridges can also work well).

Other effective options for depression include:

- Hybrid or sativa (sativa is OK only if anxiety is not a significant factor)—tinctures, edibles, and tablets (e.g., Stratos Energy tablets—low-dose THC); remember to rotate three or four products if you're taking something on a daily basis.
- 1:1/CBD:THC—tinctures and patches

In spite of the temporary improvement provided by MMJ, marijuana use on a daily basis has been found to *contribute to depression*. However, most people suffering with chronic pain have some degree of depression. If you focus on treating the underlying chronic pain condition, the depression should improve and the need for the daily use of MMJ will lessen.

HOLISTIC MEDICAL TREATMENT AND PREVENTION PROGRAM FOR DEPRESSION

Risk Factors and Causes

Depression is not well understood. The following are believed to be the most significant risk factors contributing to it:

Body: Physical (Medical) and Environmental

- Genetics—close to 50 percent of sufferers have a hereditary predisposition. Variants in the MTHFR gene, for example, could be a contributing factor.

- Candidiasis (yeast overgrowth).
- Inhalant and food allergies.
- Gut dysbiosis—an imbalance of gut bacteria that can impact mood, as 90 percent of serotonin is manufactured in the GI tract.
- Childbirth—postpartum depression.
- Female hormone dysfunction or insufficiency—PMS, perimenopause, menopause.
- Hypothyroidism.
- Hypoglycemia.
- Obesity.
- Folic acid/folate deficiency.
- Drugs and medications—Tagamet, Inderal, narcotics, benzodiazepines, birth control pills, sleeping pills, prednisone, alcohol, *marijuana.*
- Lack of exercise.
- Biochemical—low levels of the neurotransmitters serotonin and norepinephrine.
- Environmental toxicity—air pollution (decreased negative ions, increased positive ions, outgassing), heavy metal exposure (mercury, lead, cadmium).
- Decreased sunlight (seasonal affective disorder—SAD).
- Overcrowding.
- Lack of feeling grounded.

Mind: Mental and Emotional

- Distorted thinking.
- Low self-esteem.
- Grief—feelings of loss following bereavement, divorce, or retirement.
- Feelings of failure.
- Lack of stimulation.
- Addiction to work.
- Sense of helplessness.
- Lack of self-expression.
- Sense of powerlessness.
- Emotional traumas as a child: history of abuse or violence, abandonment or neglect.

Spirit: Spiritual and Social

- Lack of purpose or meaning in life.
- Feelings of isolation; lack of compassion or a committed loving relationship.
- Lack of family or social connection.
- Feeling disconnected from God/spirit.

Spiritual issues are more prominent with severe depression.

Holistic treatment along with MMJ is most effective for mild to moderate depression. Severe depression will usually require antidepressant medication, but it can be combined with many of the following physical health recommendations to enhance the therapeutic result.

Physical Health Recommendations

Air and Exposure to Nature

These factors can benefit both depression and anxiety:

- Clean air.
- Negative-ion–filled air. (Studies have shown mood benefits with levels above three thousand ions per cubic centimeter.) The highest negative-ion content air is found by seacoasts and waterfalls, on mountain tops, and in pine forests.
- Sunlight or daily exposure to full-spectrum lights.
- Beautiful natural settings—provide a sense of both grounding and relaxation.

Diet

The basic recommendation for treating depression is a diet high in complex carbohydrates such as whole grains (brown rice, barley, corn, millet, oats, and whole wheat), vegetables, beans, and fruits. These foods will boost serotonin and promote feelings of well-being. The diet should be high in protein—no less than 60 gm daily divided into three or four servings. This will help to maintain a stable blood sugar level throughout the day. In addition to food, you may want to use protein powder in diluted fruit juice or almond or soy milk, taken between meals as snacks, to meet your daily requirement.

The diet should also include red pepper, garlic, and ginger. One or two servings of cold-water fish, such as salmon or sardines, per week is recommended, as they contain high amounts of essential fatty acids (see below). Caffeine, alcohol, sugar, and refined carbohydrates (products made from white flour—bread, pasta) should be eliminated. A food-elimination diet to identify any food allergens can be very helpful.

Vitamins, Minerals, and Supplements

In many cases, natural products can have an effect on mood that is greater than or equal to that of antidepressants. Although you should start out slowly and carefully consider your unique biochemical individuality, the following amino acids, vitamins, minerals, and essential fatty acids are usually effective in treating depression:

- *Amino acids*: *DLPA (phenylalanine)* is an amino acid found to be effective for treating depression. It is a precursor (directly on the formative pathway) to norepinephrine, one of the main neurotransmitters that govern mood. The recommended dosage is to begin with 500 mg (one capsule) two times daily, on an *empty stomach with juice*. This can gradually be increased by 500 mg per day to 2 or 3 capsules, three times daily. For maximum effect, it is best to take 50 mg of *vitamin B6* at the same time, as well as *niacin*, 500 mg per day, and 1 gm of *vitamin C*. Vitamin B6 is particularly important in regulating the absorption, metabolism, and utilization of amino acids.

  L-tyrosine is an amino acid formed from phenylalanine and is one step closer to norepinephrine. The recommended dosage is exactly the same as for DLPA.

  NOTE: Glutamine is another "excitatory" amino acid that seems to combine quite well with L-tyrosine to improve its effectiveness. Some nutritional companies formulate both L-tyrosine and glutamine together. This combination capsule contains the correct ratio of both, and up to six capsules may be taken per day in divided doses on an empty stomach.

NOTE: With both DLPA and L-tyrosine, you need to be watchful for increased blood pressure, headaches, or insomnia. These side effects are indications that an excessive stimulation of the nervous system has occurred. *DO NOT take these amino acids if you are currently taking standard antidepressant medications* (the interaction between them is not well documented). *Also avoid taking these amino acids with the following conditions: phenylketonuria (PKU), hepatic cirrhosis, and melanoma.*

Like other essential amino acids, *L-tryptophan* cannot be manufactured by the body but must come directly from food or supplements. It is the building block for serotonin, the same neurotransmitter influenced by Prozac in the treatment of depression. When properly taken, tryptophan is extremely useful as a natural antidepressant as well as a sleep aid. The recommended dosage for depressive symptoms is to take 2 gm (2,000 mg) of tryptophan two or three times daily. It should be taken between meals, with fruit or juice (simple sugars) to improve its utilization. It should not be taken with a protein meal, because tryptophan competes poorly with other amino acids for absorption. To convert tryptophan to serotonin, the body must have adequate levels of folic acid, vitamin B6, magnesium, niacin, and glutamine.

The tryptophan metabolite *5-HTP*, which is much stronger than L-tryptophan, is a proven antidepressant and is available in most health food stores. The recommended dosage is 100 to 200 mg twice daily between meals.

The amino acids DLPA, L-tyrosine, and L-tryptophan should be tried one at a time. If after six weeks at a high dosage there is no improvement, then you should take a different amino acid.

Other vitamins, minerals, and supplements include:

- *B complex (containing all of the B vitamins) or B Activ (Xymogen)*: 1 capsule at breakfast and lunch daily. Postpartum depression may result from a deficiency of B6, B12, and folic acid.

- *B12*: 1,000 mcg daily, along with a weekly injection of B12, 1,000 mcg, combined with up to 5 mg of folic acid (especially for the elderly with cognitive dysfunction, or people with digestive disorders).
- *Folate (5-methyltetrahydrofolate) or 5MTHFR (Xymogen)*: 5,000 mcg (5 mg) daily for one month, then reduce to 800 mcg daily.
- *Niacinamide (vitamin B3)*: 500 mg two times daily.
- *Vitamin C*: 1,000 mg three times daily (as ascorbate or Ester-C).
- *Vitamin E*: 400 IU daily (as natural d-alpha tocopherol).
- *Magnesium or Mag Glycinate (Metagenics)*: 1,000 mg daily; necessary for the production of neurotransmitters (as glycinate or aspartate).
- *Calcium*: 1,000 mg daily (as citrate).
- *Zinc or Zinc Arginate (Metagenics)*: 30–40 mg daily.
- *Essential fatty acids (EFAs) or EPA/DHA-720 (Metagenics)*: Take 1 capsule two times daily. (The nervous system is composed of 60 percent DHA, and this EFA is essential for normal function.) For omega-6 EFAs, take evening primrose oil, 1,000 mg three times daily.
- *Phosphatidylserine (PS)*: Take 100 mg with breakfast and 200 mg with dinner (double-blind studies have proven its effectiveness with depression and insomnia).

Herbs

The therapeutic benefits of herbs often require more time than standard drugs. An advantage, however, is the safety in long-term use and the absence of reported side effects.

- *St. John's Wort (Hypericum perforatum)*: Several clinical studies have shown this herb to be as effective as standard antidepressants (amitriptyline and imipramine). The herb also has far fewer side effects. The active ingredient in St. John's wort is hypericin. The recommended dosage is 900 mg daily of 0.3 percent concentration—600 mg with breakfast and 300 mg with lunch. A trial period of one month is adequate to determine the herb's potential benefits. Do not take St. John's wort along with the DLPA and L-tyrosine if you've just started the treatment program. After four to six weeks on DLPA or L-tyrosine, you can then begin St. John's wort. Likewise, do not take St. John's wort with SSRI drugs (Prozac, Zoloft, Paxil), or with birth control pills. There is some evidence that it may accelerate the metabolism of oral contraceptives, rendering them ineffective.

- *Ginkgo biloba*: improves cerebral circulation, strengthening memory and often benefiting depression. Generally, *ginkgo* is not as effective as St. John's wort for depression, but it can be taken along with other herbs and nutrients to bolster one's overall mood. *Ginkgo biloba* should be in an extract that is standardized to contain 24 percent ginkgo flavone glycosides. The usual dose is 80–120 mg two times daily (breakfast and lunch).

- *Yohimbine*: comes from tree bark in West Africa and has been used for decades in treating male impotence or diminished libido. Recent research has indicated that yohimbine can also improve the overall effectiveness of standard antidepressant medications. In some cases, yohimbine can be used by itself to both stimulate sexual functioning and relieve mild depression in men. For mild depression and enhanced sexual functioning, take 5.4 mg of standardized yohimbine extract three times daily. A suggested trial period for this yohimbine regimen would be two to three weeks. Yohimbine can then be taken periodically as needed. *NOTE:* For some individuals, yohimbine can cause increased anxiety or uncomfortable cardiac stimulation. It should be taken under the supervision of a health professional.

- *Siberian ginseng*: Take 400 mg of a standardized extract three times daily.

- *Rosemary shampoo*: can be absorbed through the skin as well as provide aromatherapy for depression.

Exercise

The beneficial effects of regular aerobic exercise in the treatment of depression are well documented. For many years an increasing number of psychotherapists have believed that aerobic exercise, through its powerful release of endorphins, may be the most effective as well as the most economical antidepressant. However, as I mentioned in Chapter 3, a recent German study concluded that it is the endocannabinoids released during aerobic exercise, rather than endorphins, that are responsible for "runner's high."

Professional Care Therapies

- *Hormonal therapy*: Desiccated thyroid can often elicit a dramatic improvement, especially in middle-aged women. This can be true even with normal thyroid function. Lethargy, sense of cold, and fatigue are often symptoms of low thyroid function. One-half to one grain daily is a good starting dosage. DHEA can also be effective in treating depression, but the dosage should be based on blood or saliva levels of DHEA sulfate. Your physician might also check your adrenal function via cortisol/DHEA testing. This can measure maladaptive responses to stress.
- *Traditional Chinese medicine* (acupuncture and Chinese herbs) *and homeopathy* can be helpful.

The Issues in Your Tissues

Although these mental and emotional health recommendations are the same as those suggested for anxiety, they are somewhat less effective for treating depression.

Psychotherapy

The holistic psychotherapist is concerned with the presenting psychological problems as well as the life force energy or spirit of each client. What are his or her purpose and unique talents, interests, dreams, and desires in life? Where does he or she perceive a loss of love? This orientation can also be described as *spiritual psychotherapy*.

Providing the encouragement and motivation to change are the hallmarks of a skilled therapist. This can only be done by evoking the assets and gifts in each person, as well as focusing on solutions to his or her current problems. Empowerment is the essence and goal of therapy—helping clients develop their own inner resources to be a catalyst for change. Being the source of your own choices and having the capability to reinterpret any painful experience as an opportunity for learning can provide you with the energy to transform your life and cure depression. If used with a clear intention, marijuana can be a profound asset in this process of empowerment, while heightening self-awareness.

Psychotherapy is most successful when the client establishes a comfortable therapeutic rapport with the therapist. Although this connection and trust are more important than the treatment model itself, there are several psychotherapeutic options in addition to conventional psychotherapy that are helpful in treating depression. They include:

- *Cognitive/behavioral therapy (CBT)*—multiple studies have demonstrated its effectiveness in treating depression. Affirmations and imagery are an integral part of this form of therapy.
- *Mindfulness-based cognitive therapy*—one large study has shown it to be as effective as antidepressant medication, and with no adverse effects.
- *Psychosynthesis*—a holistic type of spiritual psychotherapy.
- *Hakomi therapy*—a body-centered form of psychotherapy.
- *Solution-focused/brief therapy*—a goal-oriented form of psychotherapy.
- *Spiritual psychotherapy*—described above under "Anxiety."
- *Stress-reduction techniques*—see above under "Anxiety."
- *Energy medicine*—Eye Movement Desensitization and Reprocessing (EMDR—if depression is a result of trauma), EFT, and Neurofeedback can all be helpful for treating depression. Therapies such as *Healing Touch, Therapeutic Touch, and Reiki* are all *hands-on* techniques that are helpful for treating both depression and anxiety. You'll need to find a qualified practitioner.
- *Qigong* is a moving meditation practiced by over 300 million Chinese on a daily basis that strengthens life force energy, or *chi*. It is relatively easy to learn and can be used to both treat and prevent depression and anxiety.
- Regular exposure to *sunlight* and filtered sun (twenty to thirty minutes daily) or *full-spectrum lights* that simulate sunshine can help treat depression, especially with people suffering from seasonal affective disorder. This condition is most prevalent in locations with little sunshine during the winter months.
- Soothing or stimulating *music*, or whatever sounds you resonate with, can also be helpful in treating depression.

Bodywork Therapies

A multitude of hands-on techniques can help to release deeply held or repressed emotions. Some of these methods are described as *body-centered psychotherapy* and often combine deep-tissue bodywork, such as *Rolfing*, with types of body movement, like *yoga* or *Feldenkrais*. Depression and anxiety are frequently more amenable to physical touch than to verbal therapies. These therapies are particularly important for people with a history of physical and sexual abuse or poor body image.

Spiritual and Social Health Recommendations

The most beneficial spiritual practices for treating depression are meditation, prayer, and altruism (volunteering).

Joining a support group or maintaining a connection to one is especially helpful for depressed people in strengthening their degree of social health. Working on your committed relationship with a spouse or partner can often mitigate depression.

Patient Story—**Depression**

Robert R. is a fifty-seven-year-old radiology technician with a long history of depression. He was originally diagnosed with bipolar disorder in his early thirties, shortly after a suicide attempt. He was prescribed strong antidepressants—which he said "ruined my energy, my sex life, and made me feel like a zombie" (with little or no emotion)—and Abilify.

After approximately five years on this pharmaceutical regimen, feeling hopeless and powerless, he decided to stop all of his medications and committed to healing himself. He found that smoking marijuana provided a lift, with more energy, optimism, and a greater sense of well-being. However, being prone to high levels of anxiety, he had to be careful not to smoke a strain containing too much THC. But this was prior to the legalization of medical marijuana, and detailed information about specific strains was not known.

In addition to marijuana, he modified his diet (mostly vegetarian), began taking supplements, started journaling, and did at least thirty to sixty minutes of aerobic exercise daily. He's made continual progress and today is still maintaining this same self-care regimen. The primary difference is that he now knows exactly what he's smoking or vaporizing. He generally avoids sativa strains, and prefers hybrids in a variety of forms—flower (both 50:50 hybrids and 60:40 indica-dominant strains), tinctures, edibles, tablets, and patches. He rarely misses a day of working out, feels better than he has throughout his entire adult life, and claims that "marijuana saved my life."

PART III
Fully Alive

Getting High on Life!

Introduction to Part III

Great discoveries have always encountered violent opposition from mediocre minds.

—Albert Einstein, a German-born physicist, founder
of the theory of relativity (1879–1955)

There is no question that when we're happy, we feel very good. But were you aware that nearly five decades of research in the field of psychoneuroimmunology (PNI) has documented the fact that *happiness is healthy*?

It's been repeatedly shown that our thoughts, beliefs, attitudes, and emotions can either weaken or strengthen the body's immune system, making us either more vulnerable or more resistant to disease and physical dysfunction (including the chronic pain conditions presented in Part II). The belief that you'll have to live with chronic pain for the rest of your life is *depressing*. Reinforcing this belief, the same negative thought, "I'll never get better," one that you may have been repeating to yourself multiple times a day for many months or years, *depresses immune function*.

What a startling scientific revelation! But for most of us, it's no big surprise. I'm quite sure many of you have already experienced this mind-body connection, having developed a cold on the heels of a particularly stressful event or time in your life. This might also have been the case when you experienced your first acute flare-up of what has now become a chronic condition, such as rheumatoid arthritis or fibromyalgia.

Yet in spite of its commonsense logic, this paradigm-shifting scientific discovery, with its ever-expanding body of evidence accelerating the evolution of the art and science of healing, has made barely a dent in the fortress of contemporary medical practice. Why? Greed and self-interest have seized control of the business of health care.

In 2015, America spent $3.2 *trillion* on health care, a number so large it is difficult to grasp its scale. It computes to approximately $10,000 for every one of our 320 million citizens, far exceeding any other country in the world. You might think that with such a huge expenditure we would have a very healthy population. Yet the results of a comprehensive 2015 Global Burden of Disease study show that the U.S. ranks 28 out of 188 total nations, with Iceland and Sweden ranked as the healthiest countries in the world. Nearly 86 percent of our astronomical health care expenditures ($2.7 trillion) are spent on caring for the 133 million people (45 percent of the population) suffering with at least one *chronic condition*, most of which are *preventable*.

Is it any wonder that there's been no cure for many of our most common and expensive ailments, such as cancer or heart disease, or that many effective natural remedies and cures (especially for cancer) have been outlawed by the FDA or the DEA? In many cases the practitioners who discover and promote these innovative treatments are put out of business (without any legal recourse) by these same governmental agencies.

The pharmaceutical industry is currently the second most profitable ($70 billion annually) on the planet (not far behind oil and gas), and combined with the medical and insurance industries, health care has been transformed into a thriving disease-care business with almost nothing to do with maintaining or enhancing health, or preventing disease. *The business of caring has become a lot more about business with a lot less caring.*

Conventional, allopathic, Western or "modern" medicine is based on the seventeenth-century theories of Descartes and Isaac Newton. Regarded as the *founder of modern medicine*, Descartes saw the human being as a machine with two separate parts—body (soma) and mind (psyche). Newtonian physics taught that we live in a *material universe*—all that exists is matter (invisible energy is ignored). In addition to *materialism*, the philosophical pillars of this healing art and science are composed of *reductionism* (a focus on the smallest part to understand the function and dysfunction of the whole organism) and *determinism* (if you understand how the parts work, you can accurately predict how the body will react to a drug or therapeutic modality).

For the past four hundred years this approach has evolved into our current high-tech, low-touch health care system. Conventional medicine continues to make great progress in, and is extremely effective for, treating acute and life-threatening illness, injuries, and allergic reactions, and for quickly (and temporarily) relieving discomfort (but not without risk). At times the results can be almost miraculous. For this reason, American medicine is emulated around the world. Yet a fact that is not widely recognized is that it consistently fails to cure and in most cases, prevent, a myriad of common chronic conditions, including chronic pain. When it comes to chronic disease, be it arthritis, asthma, diabetes, or high blood pressure, the stated goal of modern medicine is *management*, not *cure*!

This is why medical marijuana poses such a financial threat to the enormous profits of the pharmaceutical industry. Consider the current sales figures from opioids, sleep medications, benzodiazepines (antianxiety medications), anti-inflammatories, muscle relaxants, and anticonvulsants. Is anyone surprised that in August 2016 the FDA decided to maintain the classification of marijuana as a Schedule I drug, and just four months later the DEA recommended that CBD (a substance that has been repeatedly shown to do no harm) be placed in the same category, on equal footing with heroin and cocaine?

Modern medicine not only is ineffective at times and expensive, but can be harmful! A study published in the July 2000 issue of the *Journal of the American Medical Association (JAMA)* ranked conventional state-of-the-art medicine as the *third leading cause of death in the U.S.* (behind heart disease and cancer). The researchers used conservative *estimates* in calculating their data.

DEATHS PER YEAR

12,000—unnecessary surgery
7,000—medication errors in hospitals

20,000—other errors in hospitals

80,000—infections in hospitals

106,000—non-error negative effects of appropriately prescribed drugs

Total = 225,000 deaths per year from iatrogenic causes (i.e., caused by medical treatment)!

A year later, a group of physicians and researchers (Gary Null, PhD; Carolyn Dean MD, ND; Martin Feldman, MD; Debora Rasio, MD; and Dorothy Smith, PhD) decided to more closely scrutinize the data from the 2000 *JAMA* study and obtain more exact figures. Their research paper, entitled "Death by Medicine," appeared in *Life Extension* magazine in March 2004. From their data they concluded that conventional medicine is the *leading cause of death in the U.S.* Not surprisingly, this study was never published in a medical journal.

Their findings:

- The total number of deaths caused by conventional medicine is 783,936 per year.
- American medicine is the leading cause of death and injury in the U.S.
- By contrast, the number of deaths attributable to heart disease in 2001 was 699,697, while the number of deaths attributable to cancer was 553,251.

Table 16.1: Estimated Annual Mortality and Economic Cost of Medical Intervention		
Condition	Deaths	Cost
Adverse Drug Reactions	106,000	$12 billion
Medical error	98,000	$2 billion
Bedsores	115,000	$55 billion
Infection	88,000	$5 billion
Malnutrition	108,800	————
Outpatients	199,000	$77 billion
Unnecessary Procedures	37,136	$122 billion
Surgery-Related	32,000	$9 billion
Total	**783,936**	**$282 billion**

From these shocking statistics, it seems obvious that our current health care system is badly broken and desperately in need of change.

Conversely, integrative holistic medicine, the new *modern medicine*, is founded on *quantum physics* and the work of Albert Einstein. Regarded as the most influential physicist of the twentieth century, Einstein's theory of *relativity* (all motion must be defined relative to a frame of reference, and therefore space and time are relative, rather than absolute, concepts) was largely responsible for the development of atomic energy.

Arguably, Einstein's most significant contribution was his belief that *we live in an energy universe*, and that underneath all matter, molecules, and atoms is *invisible energy*. This energy is such a powerful force that he asserts, "The field [i.e., the environment filled with intermingling energies] *is the sole governing agency of the particle* [matter]."

The *field* includes everything from the core of your being to the outer reaches of the universe. It includes your thoughts and feelings, your diet and air quality, your relationships and faith in a higher power, as well as the energies radiating from the sun and the other planets in our solar system. *All of these energies strongly affect your physical body, and how you are affected by a specific drug or herb.* This helps to explain why patients with mild to moderate depression fare no better (sometimes worse) on antidepressants than they do with a placebo (a substance with no intrinsic therapeutic properties). Their belief that the prescription medication would help them feel better created a positive result.

Possibly the most compelling research regarding energy medicine was performed by C. W. F. McClare, a British physicist at the University of London, who compared the effect of both energy signals (e.g., thoughts, emotions, prayer, hands-on healing) and physical signals (e.g., drugs, hormones) on cells. He discovered that *energy signals were one hundred times more efficient than physical signals*!

Einstein's quantum physics and his theory of an *energy universe* have profound implications for the practice of medicine, but unfortunately they have not yet changed the way most doctors diagnose and treat their patients.

• • •

Doctors who serve as teachers as well as healers, and provide in-depth self-care education, do not generate sufficient revenue to satisfy the gluttonous financial appetite of the medical/pharmaceutical industry. Cure and prevention are not profitable. But from my forty-five years as a family physician, I can categorically state that *self-care is a far more effective, economical, and empowering approach for treating chronic pain and disease than our current health care system.*

So miraculous is the mind-body connection that researchers in the field of psychoneuroimmunology have concluded that the immune system is in fact a *circulating nervous system* mediated by neurotransmitters (i.e., substances that transmit nerve impulses across a synapse). I've previously mentioned that THC promotes the release of the neurotransmitter dopamine. This substance has been defined as the kick-ass chemical in your brain that makes you feel and do happy things . . . whatever they may be. Very simply, *dopamine creates happiness.*

Knowledge is power. In Part III, using *cannabis as a facilitator in a potentially life-changing holistic healing process*, I am providing you with several safe and practical options for gaining greater *self-knowledge*, which equates with *self-power*.

After engaging in these practices on a consistent basis for at least three months, you will have much *less pain*; develop a greater appreciation for the intimate connection between your body, mind, and soul; heighten awareness of your limiting and creative thoughts as well as your painful and joyful emotions; and learn to more consciously strengthen your immune function.

You will become much better acquainted with your true self, the *heart of you* that you may have kept hidden through most of adolescence and may have had only a few brief glimpses during your entire adult life. With a clear intention, you will be creating the life of your dreams, along with a better understanding of who you are, why you're here, where your heart is guiding you, and how to experience a depth of happiness you've never known. In short, you will become more *fully alive*!

Chapter 16

Cannabis as a Sacred Herb

Joy is the infallible sign of the presence of God.

—Pierre Teilhard de Chardin, a French philosopher
and Jesuit priest (1881–1955)

*F*ully alive is living a life filled with passion, purpose, and play! This
and the following chapter will provide you with a practical personalized guide for experiencing such a life, with cannabis as a facilitator,
not a constant companion.

There is no emotion more therapeutic for creating optimal health
and happiness than *love*. Holistic physicians believe that *unconditional
love (UL) is life's most powerful healer*, and that the *perceived loss of love
is our greatest health risk*.

The only problem with this concept is that the vast majority of us
have only a vague idea what this term means. I'm sure we received a
strong dose of UL as newborns and infants, but who remembers? We
may still have a cellular memory of the feeling, but for many adults, our
dogs provide the greatest and most consistent source of UL. (I admit
I'm a dog guy, but I've been told by many cat owners that they feel lots
of love from their feline friends as well.)

I'm still working on it, but my latest definition of unconditional love
is *total acceptance of yourself exactly as you are, and the realization that
we are all one with each other, with all of Earth's inhabitants, and with
God*. Healing is a process, one in which progress is measured by your

capacity to give and receive love. *The art of loving is our life's work, and the primary purpose for our presence on Earth.*

LOVE HEALS! We know that to be true on an intuitive level, and science has helped to reinforce this universal truth. But most of us need guidance in becoming highly skilled caretakers of our body, mind, emotions, heart, and soul. The practice of holistic healing is not a one-size-fits-all approach, as is conventional medical practice, in which the diagnosis determines the treatment. This is the primary reason Western medicine consistently *fails to cure nearly all chronic conditions.* In this and the following chapters, I'm providing several options for you to include in the creation of your own personalized self-care training program.

Chronic pain is a messenger alerting you to the need for more nurturing attention to specific aspects of your life. The issues in the tissues of the dysfunctional body part are often those that you've been consciously or unconsciously avoiding for most of your life. The shingles virus served as a harsh reminder to me that I had more work to do. I'm not saying it's easy to confront feelings of anger, sadness, guilt, shame, or the fear of rejection, but it's not as arduous a process as you might think. Emotional pain hurts, but *if you don't feel it, you can't heal it.*

As you embark on this life-changing journey, *cannabis can serve as a facilitator and assist you in navigating through your uncharted interior landscape.* It will help to empower you and accelerate the healing process. However, once the door to higher consciousness is opened, with consistent practice cannabis is no longer necessary to keep it open. But when used on occasion as a sacred heart-opening, soul-awakening herb, it can help take you to new heights of self-awareness and self-love.

There's no question that it's a formidable challenge to learn to love unconditionally, particularly to love yourself. That's especially true while living in our highly judgmental, competitive, materialistic, money- and ego-driven world, one in which self-worth is often measured by net worth. However, regardless of the difficulty you may experience, *giving and receiving love as your highest priority and greatest value in life,* while *appreciating and accepting yourself exactly as you are,* will set you free from the constraints imposed by our largely head-ruled society.

I'm not suggesting that you relinquish your brilliant thoughts and creative ideas, or that you isolate yourself from the world you live in, only that you lessen your attachment to its values and listen more attentively to your *heart*. Spiritual teachers have referred to the heart as the *seat of the soul—the home of your true self or God-self*. By more equitably balancing mind and heart, you are better able to clarify your needs and desires, make healthier choices, and embrace your passions. When it is used with intention, I've found cannabis to be immensely helpful in maintaining this delicate balance.

The human heart is in fact far more than a pump. Researchers at the HeartMath Institute in California have determined that the physiology and nerve centers of the heart are so complex and active that they constitute a "brain" all on their own, termed a *"mini-brain."* We now know that the heart contains cells that produce and release norepinephrine and dopamine, neurotransmitters once thought to be produced only by the brain and by ganglia outside the heart. Even more remarkable is the discovery that the heart produces oxytocin, the "love hormone"—in concentrations that are as high as those in the brain.

The energy conveyed by *cannabis is both medicinal and mystical,* which is most evident with its impact on the heart. Parts I and II have provided you with a wealth of information on the use of cannabis as a medicine, primarily for physical pain relief. In Part III you will learn to apply the *mystical heart chakra–opening properties of the herb to heal the deeper emotional and spiritual pain underlying all physical pain.*

The word *mystical* is defined as:

- inspiring a sense of spiritual mystery, awe, and fascination;
- concerned with the soul or the spirit, rather than with material things;
- having a spiritual *meaning* or reality that is neither apparent to the senses nor obvious to the intelligence;
- involving an individual's direct subjective communion with God or ultimate reality.

The word *sacred* is defined as "connected with God" and is often used as a synonym for *mystical* or *holy*. From this perspective, health is a *state of wholeness and balance of body, mind, and spirit.*

The American Board of Integrative Holistic Medicine (ABIHM) defines holistic or optimal health as the *unlimited and unimpeded free flow of life force energy through your body, mind, and spirit*. Although Western medicine has so far been unable to prove the existence of life force energy (and therefore ignores it), just as with the concept of *gravity*, we know it's there by observing its effect on the material world.

Nearly every ancient culture and health care discipline has been based on the concept of life force energy. Known as *chi* (Chinese), *ki* (Japanese), *pranna* (Sanskrit/Ayurveda; *chakra* = energy center), *chai* (Hebrew), and the *tao* (Taoism), holistic practitioners call it *bioenergy* or *unconditional love*.

Life force energy is responsible for the self-healing mechanisms inherent in the human body. One of the most consistently efficient methods I've found for strengthening this vital life force is the *intentional use of cannabis*. I believe this occurs as a result of its *heart chakra–opening* properties.

Recent research has revealed that the heart's electrical power is forty to sixty times greater than that of the brain, while its magnetic power radiates out at five thousand to six thousand times greater than that from the brain. This means that the heart is fully alive with a consciousness embracing the essence or seat of the soul, and an intelligence that in many ways surpasses that of the brain. It also bestows on the heart a remarkable therapeutic capacity for healing our body, mind, emotions, and soul. Cannabis helps to heighten your awareness of this powerful inner healer, in addition to the emotional issues contributing to your pain, not through the mind, but by facilitating *felt perceptions* and *vibratory knowing*.

To derive the full potential of this unique medicinal and mystical plant, the energy of cannabis must be used in a way that harnesses its basic properties to promote holistic health. When used appropriately, it can have a profound healing and enlightening effect. For this reason, sects within Tibetan Buddhism, Hinduism, Taoism, Sufism, and a variety of other religious groups have included cannabis in their spiritual practices for several millennia.

Throughout the remainder of this and the following chapter, I will present a variety of self-care practices that can enhance the flow of life force energy through your body, mind, emotions, relationships, and spirit. They will provide you with valuable tools for gaining greater peace of mind and self-acceptance, a sense of purpose, and the self-esteem required to take the risks and proceed on your healing path, as well as enjoying more play and passion in your life.

If you commit to diligently practicing one or more of these disciplines, you will significantly reinforce and enhance the improvement you may have experienced from the combination of MMJ and holistic medicine recommendations in Part II, and possibly permanently relieve your physical pain, cure your disease, and heal your life.

REMEMBER THE SABBATH DAY, TO KEEP IT HOLY.

One of the Ten Commandments—Exodus 20:8

I've been using cannabis on a regular basis, once or twice a week, since 1966. For the past thirty years my personal use has been largely limited to integrating it into the Sabbath ritual and using it with intention as a *sacred herb*. According to most rabbis, more so than Yom Kippur (the Day of Atonement [At-one-ment] and Forgiveness—a day of fasting), the Sabbath day is considered the holiest day of the year, even though it occurs weekly. As one of the Ten Commandments, it stands on equal footing with "Thou shalt not" kill or steal or commit adultery. That certainly gives us a clear picture of the importance of the Sabbath from God's perspective.

In addition to prayer and the absence of work, the ritual begins by welcoming the Sabbath with the lighting of candles, followed by *wine*, the great facilitator for quickly relaxing and more fully enjoying the gifts of the Sabbath. Wine is prescribed at least four times throughout the Sabbath day. My problem in strictly adhering to tradition is that wine makes me sleepy, and although relaxed, I'm then not particularly energized and joyful. Alcohol is, after all, pharmacologically classified as a *depressant*.

Never having been a letter-of-the-law kind of guy, I've always been more interested in meaning, purpose, and the *spirit* of the law. In celebrating the Sabbath, it's obvious that the wine serves as a natural substance to quickly alter your consciousness, help you relax, free you from the cares and concerns of the workweek, encourage you to devote yourself to enjoying life's pleasures, and assist you in connecting with God. This is a day to stop *doing* and fully appreciate the delight of simply *being* alive. Singing and dancing are highlights of a traditional *Shabbat* (Hebrew for "Sabbath") celebration. It is a particularly good day to practice *gratitude* and contemplate the *blessings* you share with those you love.

Rabbi Levi Brackman believes that "the Sabbath is mindfulness." He is the founder of Judaism in the Foothills, in Evergreen, Colorado, and teaches a yearlong program called Health and Wellness Judaism. It focuses on the intersection of ancient practices in Judaism and current health and social science—specifically, peer-reviewed academic research that relates to religious practices and tenets. In describing the Sabbath, he said, "It dawned on me that you're not supposed to focus on the week that went by, you're not supposed to focus on the week that's coming—it's kind of this island of time when you focus on the present."

In keeping with the spirit of this holy day, I substitute another natural substance, one that opens my heart and heightens my awareness, triggering feelings of *relaxed vitality*, *present moment awareness*, and *happiness*.

Marijuana alters my consciousness, empowering me to become more deeply aware of sensing, feeling, moving, and thinking. It *lightens* my load, allowing me to relax, be silly, laugh, play, go with the flow, and let go of stress and the seriousness of life; *inspires* my mind with vivid and creative ideas and visions; *opens* my heart, filling it with compassion and forgiveness, stimulating great sex and deep intimacy, strengthening acceptance and connection to my true self/soul; *soothes* my soul by awakening to the realization that I am, and everyone else is, a child of God, a unique spiritual being sharing a human experience, and creating a sense of oneness with All-That-Is; *magnifies* my gratitude to our Creator who has blessed us with this opportunity to play in the field of time and space; *reminds* me that it's all good and it's all God; and overall, *generates in me a profound love of life.*

I believe this is what God had in mind with the commandment "Remember the Sabbath day, to keep it holy." This state of holiness and happiness, which at times is pure *bliss*, is what *getting high* means to me. In short, it feels wonderful! And if that's not enough pleasure, to complete the Sabbath evening celebration, Orthodox Jews prescribe having intercourse with your spouse or partner on Friday nights.

There are *blessings* recited before each glass of wine, each meal, and for me, before vaporizing *marijuana*. Thanks to a physician friend and colleague, I now have a Hebrew blessing for this sacred medicinal herb: *Baruch ahtah Adonai, elohaynu melech ha'olam, boray who ha essev.* "Blessed art thou O Lord our God, King of the Universe, who has blessed us with the grass." With this blessing I set an *intention*, and the Sabbath almost immediately becomes a *mystical experience*.

The traditional *Shabbat* is celebrated from sundown on Friday, beginning with the ritual described above, to Saturday sunset. Its conclusion is marked by a brief *Havdalah* (Hebrew for "separation") ceremony. This ritual involves lighting a special Havdalah candle with several wicks, blessing a cup of wine, and smelling sweet spices. Following Havdalah, we wish each other *Shavua Tov*—"a good week!"

Although this traditional Sabbath lasts for twenty-four hours, it can be observed in whatever way feels most meaningful to you, and whenever it works best for you. If time is limited, it need not be an entire day. Three or four hours can work quite well, but I do suggest that at least half of this abbreviated Sabbath should be *alone* time. And it's best to observe on the same day and time each week in order to plan and schedule it. I've also found that vaporizing once or twice a week in conjunction with this holy day is far more effective as a spiritual medicine than using marijuana on a daily basis (as I did for nearly nine months during the acute post-herpetic pain phase of shingles).

I like to observe the tradition on Friday nights with my wife, family, and friends; and then spend three or four hours alone on Saturday morning. When it's observed in this way, I experience the Sabbath as *holy*, a day devoted to God or Spirit, to nurturing oneself and loved ones, and to having fun. I've never considered myself a religious person, but experiencing Sabbath with cannabis is a highly pleasurable and healing spiritual practice for me.

I recommend using this sacred herb as an essential component of your spiritual practice of Sabbath once a week, preferably on a day when you're not working, for a *minimum* of two to three hours. It's best to use a sativa-dominant strain (either 60:40 or 70:30; if anxiety is one of your issues, then a 50:50 strain is preferable), to benefit from the psychoactive effect, and to be alone with no distractions, such as a computer (other than for writing or journaling), TV, or phone (don't answer the phone).

My personal preference is to vaporize, because it begins working right away, and my intention can sometimes become clearer immediately *after* getting high. It is also effective to use a tincture, edible, or tablet, but I would suggest waiting until you begin feeling the psychoactive effect before proceeding with your spiritual practice. The effect is enhanced even further if you have an empty stomach, except for possibly a green drink or protein shake.

Begin your Sabbath (you can call it whatever you want, but this is your *sacred time*) with an *intention*: What are you seeking (e.g., peace of mind, less pain, more direction with a project you're working on, etc.)? What is it that you'd like help with from your spirit guides? What question do you need answered (e.g., "What do I need to learn from this pain, so I can let it go?" "What is the next step in my spiritual growth?" "What am I here to do?" "How can I best serve?" "Who am I?")? Relaxing or inspirational music, meditation, prayer, a journal or notebook to record your thoughts and feelings, a walk in nature, yoga, qigong, or any other practice meaningful to you can be included as part of your Sabbath ritual.

Remember, this is an *island of time* in which you focus on the present moment: What are you feeling, visualizing, hearing, thinking? This oasis of a few hours of present moment awareness is a nurturing gift you're giving yourself each week.

With my solo Sabbath ritual, after setting an intention and getting high, I first do a twenty-minute meditation that I learned from reading and practicing *The Presence Process,* by Michael Brown. This book serves as a superb guide to *present moment awareness.* The daily practice (the rest of the week I do this meditation without getting high, as Brown recommends) begins with the following mantra: *I am, here now, in this.* The words are not spoken verbally but are focused on in conjunction with each connected breath (i.e., no pause at the end of each inhalation and exhalation)—*I* (inhale) *am* (exhale), *here* (inhale) *now* (exhale), *in* (inhale) *this* (exhale).

Next, I recite the Invocation of the Cardinal Directions, which I learned from Richard Sandore, a physician shaman, during the first of three training sessions with him in July 2003. This helps to create a sacred space and combines both Native North and South American tribal traditions. The words *our* and *we* are used, since the Invocation is typically part of a *group* ceremony. I recommend doing it alone several times to feel comfortable with it and to more fully appreciate its value, before inviting others to join you. If your preference is to keep doing it alone, as I typically do, you can visualize your loved ones included within the energy field you're generating.

As I recite, I turn to face each of the four directions, with arms raised, hands at shoulder level, and palms facing away from me (to receive the energy of that direction), or if you prefer, your arms can hang at your side. For Pachamama (Earth goddess of the Incas), palms face down, and for Great Spirit (Native American term for God), they face up.

As I complete each direction, I raise my voice as I recite the word *Hayaya*. This is Quechua (the language still spoken by descendants of the Incas in the Andes of South America), and although there is no known translation, it essentially means "So be it!" I also shake a Native American rattle for added emphasis.

Following and often during the recitation of this Invocation is when *the magic of this mystical herb begins* to emerge. Visions related to your intention and answers to your questions may come to you—a direct communication from your heart/soul.

INVOCATION OF THE CARDINAL DIRECTIONS

South

To the Winds of the South, Kunti Wayra. Great Serpent, Mother of the Waters, come and be with us. Sachamama, Hantun Amaru, come be with us, wrap your coils of light around us and guide us on our journeys of healing. Great Healer, come be with us and teach us your ways. Teach us to shed our past, to shed all of our old beliefs, all of our old ways of thinking that no longer serve us. Sachamama, teach us to shed these all at once, as an act of love, and as an act of power, as you shed your skin. Hayaya, Sachamama.

West

To the Winds of the West, Chinchay Wayra. Otorongo, Great Jaguar, Mother-Sister Jaguar, come be with us and teach us your ways. Otorongo, Hantun Otorongo, teach us to walk softly and stealthily upon the mother. And teach us to walk without fear. Rainbow Jaguar, teach us to release all of our fears, to walk fearlessly through this life, and to fearlessly leap from this world to all of those worlds beyond. And Otorongo, teach us to be warriors, luminous warriors, warriors without need for enemies in this world or any of those worlds beyond. Hayaya, Otorongo.

North

To the Winds of the North, Anti Wayra. Kuraq Akullipaq, Ancient Ones, you who have come before, you who have yet to come, you who are the keepers of our children's children, come be with us and teach us your ways. Come sit by us, walk next to us, and lend us the knowledge you know, the mysteries you've uncovered. Huanacautti, Rainbow Prince, come teach us the ways of power. And Kenti, Sewarkenti, Hummingbird, come fly next to us and whisper in our ears your sweet song of knowledge. Hayaya, Ancient Ones.

East

To the Winds of the East, Chollo Wayra. Brother Eagle, Sister Condor, come be with us and teach us your ways. Apuchin Apu Kondor, Hantun Kondor, come open your wings of light around our hearts, open our hearts that we may see. Lend us your vision that we may see beyond our horizons. Sister Condor, you who flies high above the mountains, you who lives above the clouds, come teach us to soar, teach us to open our wings and soar to those places we've never dreamed of going to before. Hayaya, Sister Condor.

Pachamama

Pachamama, Santa Taita Pachamama, Pachamamita, Loving Mother, Mother Earth. Mother, you who have never left us, you who will never leave us, you who holds us so tenderly all of the time. We thank you for nourishing and nurturing us, for holding us, and for all of the light and love and beauty you bring into our lives. And we thank you for the company of all of your children, those that walk and those that crawl, those that fly and those that swim, the two-legged, the three-legged, and the multi-legged, the furred, the feathered, and the finned. And Pachamama, tell us what we can do for you to return the love you give to us. We love you, Pachamama. Hayaya, Pachamama.

Great Spirit

Inti Taita, Father Sun, Mama Killa, Grandmother Moon, Illiatitsa, Wirachocha, Waykan Tanka, Tankashala, Great Spirit. You who are known by a thousand names, yet you who are the nameless one. You who are in the north, the south, the east, and the west. You who are in the plant people, the stone people, our star brothers and sisters, our mother, and each and every one of us. We thank you for giving us this opportunity to play in the field of time and space. Be with us, guide us on our journeys, and teach us, teach us always, always, always to manifest the You within each and every one of us, and to share that gift with those we share our lives with. Hayaya, Great Spirit.

Center

You are now within the center of the universe you've assembled. This is recognized with a brief moment of silence to feel the space you've created.

If your preference is to engage in a sacred cannabis ceremony with others, the International Church of Cannabis opened its doors in Denver on April 20, 2017. Headquarters of Elevation Ministries, a nonprofit religious organization, it claims cannabis as its primary sacrament. The goal of its members, known as Elevationists, is "to create the best version of themselves," and they believe cannabis accelerates and deepens that process. As legalization expands, I expect many more people will be using cannabis as a sacred herb and similar groups will be established in other states.

In the remainder of Part III, I will present several holistic health practices that you can choose to include in your Sabbath ritual while you're high, as well as engage in daily without cannabis.

Chapter 17

What Is Your Dream?

The world only exists in your eyes—your conception of it. You can make it as big or as small as you want to.

   —F. Scott Fitzgerald, an American novelist (1896–1940)

Follow your bliss and the universe will open doors where there were only walls.

   —Joseph Campbell, an American mythologist, writer, and lecturer (1904–1987)

Concerning all acts of initiative (and creation), there is one elementary truth, the ignorance of which kills countless ideas and splendid plans: that the moment one definitely commits oneself, then Providence moves too. All kinds of things occur to help one that would never otherwise have occurred. . . . Whatever you can do, or dream you can do, begin it. Boldness has genius, power and magic in it. Begin it now.

   —Johann Wolfgang von Goethe, a German writer and statesman (1749–1832)

Each of us is creating our own reality, guided by our thoughts, beliefs, visions, and attitudes. How thrilling a journey it has been for the past thirty years to *consciously* create the life of my dreams. It hasn't always been smooth sailing, but for the most part, I've stayed true to the mission of transforming health care by establishing a new specialty based on the belief that *love is life's most powerful healer*. For one of the elders of the baby boomers, who protested the war in Vietnam in Washington, DC, in 1968 (my first year in medical school) carrying a sign, *Make Love Not War*, my life has been a dream come true!

What's your wildest dream? It may be something that you've dismissed because you believed it would *never be possible to have, be, or do* whatever it is you've envisioned for yourself. But suppose while enjoying your Sabbath or after getting high, you let go of your overprotective and limiting mind and surrendered to your heart. Picture in your mind's eye what you'd love your life to look like, even though you may not have a clue how it could possibly happen. *Trust* that your heart will guide you in the direction of the most fulfilling, enriching, and nurturing vision.

I realize this poses a challenge for most of us. It's not the way you normally do things. But the more calculated risks you take, the greater will be your capacity to trust that the outcome will benefit you in some way. If you remain committed to your goal in spite of the setbacks (see them as valuable lessons), you'll find that ultimately you will manifest something quite close to what you envisioned, although it most likely will not occur in the way you expected or as quickly as you wanted.

The combination of *desire, belief, expectancy, persistence, and patience is a winning formula for manifestation*. Unless you are continually meeting with formidable obstacles (a message that your vision needs some modification), the process of living your dream can flow almost effortlessly. It doesn't mean there won't be setbacks, but none of them will prove to be insurmountable, and a solution is often found relatively soon. This is especially true if your goal will benefit others.

Even if it's just for three hours a week, that's more than enough time for cannabis to serve as a masterful facilitator in the co-creation (you, along with your higher self/soul, spirit guides, and God) and evolution of the blueprint for the life of your dreams.

After you've vaporized and possibly recited the Invocation of the Cardinal Directions, the process of heightening self-, soul-, or heart-awareness can comprise the bulk of your Sabbath ritual. You will always learn something of great value while in this altered state. Your heart opens, fear diminishes, and trust that your life is unfolding perfectly expands. You might also feel a deep sense of gratitude for everything and everyone in your life (they're all your teachers, especially those who repeatedly push your buttons).

Each of us is unique and no two people will react exactly the same way. If this is a new experience for you, I understand the fear of the unknown, but if it is used appropriately there is nothing to fear from the psychoactive (THC) properties of marijuana. Quite the opposite is true. It can be a highly nurturing and enlivening experience.

The quality of your experience while you're high is dependent on several variables, including the specific strain of cannabis, the setting in which it's being used, your emotional state before partaking, and the clarity of your intention. An intention is the compass for keeping you on track and directing you along your healing path. For the purpose of clarifying your dream, your intention might be: *To envision the life of my dreams.* Or more specifically (this is preferable): *To relieve my chronic pain; to create a vibrantly healthy body; to work at a job that I find fulfilling and fun; to find my soulmate; to take the next step in my healing process and have the courage to confront and feel my emotional pain.*

Getting high might also serve as an opportunity for you to listen to the voice and possibly the anguish of your largely ignored and neglected *inner child*, the part of you with unmet needs. Perhaps you didn't receive the love, nurturing attention, and playtime you most needed when you were younger. To a great extent your current physical pain may be associated with the deep emotional wounds you experienced as a child. Your parents may not have done such a great job (they did the best they could), so you are, in essence, *re-parenting your inner child.* In this case, a broad intention might be: *To heal my inner child*—with more specifics to follow as you heighten self-awareness. *This pact for healing your wounded inner child is the most direct path I know for practicing exceptional self-care and relieving your pain.*

Your desire to relieve pain is quite clear. But when the pain is gone (or on the way out), what would you like your life to look like? What are some of your passions that have for many years lain dormant? What other aspects of your life have you been neglecting? You can clarify some of these questions, while measuring your current state of holistic health, by completing the Fully Alive Questionnaire (FAQ), and then using these results to identify aspects of your life that need more attention and *intention*. This information will help you to eventually *get high on life* without the use of marijuana or any other mind-altering substance.

To measure progress, most patients find it helpful to re-take the FAQ following a minimum of a three-month commitment to the holistic medical treatment program for their specific condition, which also includes the practices described in this chapter.

FULLY ALIVE QUESTIONNAIRE

Answer the questions in each section below and total your score. Each response will be a number from 0 to 5. Please refer to the frequency described within the parentheses (e.g., "2 to 3 times/week") when answering questions about an *activity*—for example, "Do you maintain a healthy diet?" However, when the question refers to an *attitude* or an *emotion* (most of the Mind and Spirit questions)—for example, "Do you have a sense of humor?"—the response is more subjective and less exact, and you should refer to the terms describing the frequency, such as *often* or *daily*, but not to the numbered frequencies in parentheses.

> 0 = Never or almost never (once a year or less)
> 1 = Seldom (2 to 12 times/year)
> 2 = Occasionally (2 to 4 times/month))
> 3 = Often (2 to 3 times/week)
> 4 = Regularly (4 to 6 times/week)
> 5 = Daily

BODY: Physical and Environmental Health

1. Do you maintain a healthy diet (low fat, low sugar, fresh fruits, grains, and vegetables)? ____

2. Is your water intake adequate (at least $\frac{1}{2}$ oz/lb of body weight—160 lbs = 80 oz—or 10 gm/450 gm of body weight)? ____

3. Are you within 20 percent of your ideal body weight? ____

4. Do you feel physically attractive? ____

5. Do you fall asleep easily and sleep soundly? ____

6. Do you awaken in the morning feeling well rested? ____

7. Do you have more than enough energy to meet your daily responsibilities? ____

8. Are your five senses acute? ____

9. Do you take time to experience sensual pleasure? ____

10. Do you schedule regular massage or deep-tissue body work? ____

11. Does your sexual relationship feel gratifying? ____

12. Do you engage in regular physical workouts (lasting at least 20 minutes)? ____

13. Do you have good endurance or aerobic capacity? ____

14. Do you breathe abdominally for at least a few minutes daily? ____

15. Do you maintain physically challenging goals? ____

16. Are you physically strong? ____

17. Do you do some stretching exercises? ____

18. Are you free of chronic aches, pains, ailments, and diseases? ____

19. Do you have regular effortless bowel movements? ____

20. Do you understand the causes of your chronic physical problems? ____

21. Are you free of any drug or alcohol dependency?   ____

22. Do you live and work in a healthy environment with respect to clean air, water, and indoor pollution?   ____

23. Do you feel energized or empowered by nature?   ____

24. Do you feel a strong connection with and appreciation for your body, your home, and your environment?   ____

25. Do you have an awareness of life-energy or *qi*?   ____

TOTAL BODY SCORE: _____

MIND: Mental and Emotional Health

1. Do you have specific goals in your personal and professional life? ____

2. Do you have the ability to concentrate for extended periods of time?   ____

3. Do you use visualization or mental imagery to help you attain your goals or enhance your performance?   ____

4. Do you believe it is possible to change?   ____

5. Can you meet your financial needs and desires?   ____

6. Is your outlook basically optimistic?   ____

7. Do you give yourself more supportive messages than critical messages?   ____

8. Does your job utilize all of your greatest talents?   ____

9. Is your job enjoyable and fulfilling?   ____

10. Are you willing to take risks or make mistakes in order to succeed?   ____

11. Are you able to adjust beliefs and attitudes as a result of learning from painful experiences?   ____

12. Do you have a sense of humor?   ____

13. Do you maintain peace of mind and tranquillity?   ____

14. Are you free from a strong need for control or the need to be right?   ____

15. Are you able to fully experience your painful feelings such as fear, anger, sadness, and hopelessness?   ____

16. Are you aware of and able to safely express fear?   ____

17. Are you aware of and able to safely express anger?   ____

18. Are you aware of and able to safely express sadness or to cry?   ____

19. Are you accepting of all your feelings?   ____

20. Do you engage in meditation, contemplation, or psychotherapy to better understand your feelings?   ____

21. Is your sleep free from disturbing dreams?   ____

22. Do you explore the symbolism and emotional content of your dreams?   ____

23. Do you take the time to let your guard down and relax, or make time for activities that constitute the abandon or absorption of play?   ____

24. Do you experience feelings of exhilaration? ____

25. Do you enjoy high self-esteem? ____

TOTAL MIND SCORE: _____

SPIRIT: Spiritual and Social Health

1. Do you actively commit time to your spiritual life? ____

2. Do you take time for prayer, meditation, or reflection? ____

3. Do you listen and act upon your intuition? ____

4. Are creative activities a part of your work or leisure time? ____

5. Do you take risks? ____

6. Do you have faith in God, spirit guides, or angels? ____

7. Are you free from anger toward God? ____

8. Are you grateful for the blessings in your life? ____

9. Do you take walks, garden, or have contact with nature? ____

10. Are you able to let go of your attachment to specific outcomes and embrace uncertainty? ____

11. Do you observe a day of rest completely away from work, dedicated to nurturing yourself and your family? ____

12. Can you let go of self-interest in deciding the best course of action for a given situation? ____

13. Do you feel a sense of purpose? ____

14. Do you make time to connect with young children, either your own or someone else's? ____

15. Are playfulness and humor important to you in your daily life? ____

16. Do you have the ability to forgive yourself and others? ____

17. Have you demonstrated the willingness to commit to a marriage or comparable long-term relationship? ____

18. Do you experience intimacy, besides sex, in your committed relationships? ____

19. Do you confide in or speak openly with one or more close friends? ____

20. Do you or did you feel close with your parents? ____

21. If you have experienced the loss of a loved one, have you fully grieved that loss? ____

22. Has your experience of pain enabled you to grow spiritually? ____

23. Do you go out of your way or give your time to help others? ____

24. Do you feel a sense of belonging to a group or community? ____

25. Do you experience unconditional love? ____

TOTAL SPIRIT SCORE: _____

TOTAL BODY, MIND, SPIRIT SCORE: _____

Health Scale

325–375	Optimal Health: FULLY ALIVE
275–324	Excellent Health
225–274	Good Health
175–224	Fair Health
125–174	Below Average Health
75–124	Poor Health
Less than 75	Extremely Unhealthy: SURVIVING

THE MIND-BODY CONNECTION

The greatest discovery of any generation is that human beings can alter their lives by altering the attitudes of their minds.

> —Albert Schweitzer, a French-German theologian,
> philosopher, physician, and medical missionary
> (1875–1965)

In his classic treatise *The Science of Mind*, noted spiritual teacher Ernest Holmes wrote: "Health and sickness are largely externalizations of our dominant mental and spiritual states. A normal healthy mind reflects itself in a healthy body, and conversely, an abnormal mental state expresses its corresponding condition in some physical condition." At the time Holmes wrote those words, in the mid-1920s, modern science was far behind him in understanding how *our thoughts directly influence our physical health.*

Socrates, a Greek philosopher considered one of the founders of Western philosophy (lived during the fourth century BC), stated that *an unexamined life is not worth living.* Based on today's research in the field of behavioral medicine, I would paraphrase his statement to say, *the unexamined belief is not worth believing in.* Yet most of us have never taken the time to reflect on the beliefs we hold. We therefore remain unaware of the extent to which they govern our behavior, and how effectively they are currently serving us or affecting our state of well-being. Do most of your core beliefs, the majority of which you've held since childhood, reflect the truth of who you are today? If not, you can choose to replace them with those that do.

Today a growing body of evidence indicates that it is our predominant, habitual beliefs that determine the thoughts we primarily think, and supports the accuracy of Ernest Holmes's conclusions. I consider it one of the most exciting developments in the field of medicine in recent decades—the scientific verification that *our physical health is directly influenced by our thoughts, beliefs, and emotions.*

While Eastern systems of medicine, such as traditional Chinese medicine and Ayurveda, have for centuries recognized these facts and stressed the importance of a harmonious connection between body and mind, in the West this mind-body connection did not begin to be acknowledged until research conducted in the 1970s and '80s conclusively revealed the ability of thoughts, emotions, and attitudes to influence our body's immune functions. In fact, many of the scientists exploring this relatively new field of psychoneuroimmunology (PNI) have concluded that *there is no separation between mind and body.*

Scientists now commonly speak of the mind's ability to control the body. In large part, this belief is the result of the scientific discovery of "messenger" molecules known as *neuropeptides*, chemicals that communicate our thoughts, emotions, attitudes, and beliefs to every cell in our body. In practical terms, this means that all of us are capable of either weakening or strengthening our immune system according to how we think and feel. Moreover, scientists have also proven that these messages can originate not only in the brain but from every cell in our body. As a result of such studies, scientists now conclude that the immune system actually functions as a *circulating nervous system* that is actively and acutely attuned to our every thought and emotion.

Once you accept the fact that there is an ongoing, instant, and intimate communication occurring between your mind and your body via the mechanisms of neuropeptides, you can also see that *the person best qualified to direct that communication in your own life is you.* Learning how to do so effectively can enable you to become your own twenty-four-hour-a-day healer by becoming more conscious of your thoughts and emotions and managing them better, to improve all areas of your health. This awareness, coupled with the belief that *anything's possible*, can provide you with the opportunity to have, to do, and to be whatever you want.

The first step in this process is acknowledging that you can no longer afford to continue feeding yourself the same limiting messages you most likely have been conditioned to accept since early childhood. This is especially true of someone who was continually shamed by a highly critical parent. The belief that "I'm a bad boy (or girl)," and not deserving of love, doesn't just disappear when you become an adult.

Scientists estimate that the average person has approximately fifty thousand thoughts each day; yet 95 percent of them are the same as the ones the person had the day before. Typically such thoughts are not only subconscious but often critical and limiting. For example: "I'm going to have to learn to live with this pain for the rest of my life." "I'll never get better." "I'll always be dependent on these narcotics to relieve the pain." "There's nothing more that can be done for me."

When you're hearing messages like these repeated many times during the course of a typical day, it's easy to understand why for most people with chronic pain, *fear, anger, hopelessness, sadness, and depression* may become their predominant feelings. These *painful emotions not only weaken your immune system but also contribute to increasing your physical pain*. However, *by consciously taking control of your thoughts and recognizing how they govern your behavior, you can dramatically change your life and heal your dis-ease*. You will gain the freedom to think, feel, and believe as you choose, thereby flooding your body's cells with positive, life-affirming messages capable of contributing to your optimal health.

Learning how to free yourself from such distorted and illogical thinking patterns, often rooted in the past, and to create a life filled with passion, purpose, and play, one that you love living, is the primary objective of the *self-care* approaches presented in the remainder of this chapter. You can begin practicing them immediately to heal your mind, your emotional body, and your relationships, along with your backache, migraines, or any other chronic pain condition.

BELIEFS/GOALS/AFFIRMATIONS

We are what we think. All that we are arises with our thoughts. With our thoughts, we make the world.

—Buddha

Anyone who has never made a mistake has never tried anything new.

—Albert Einstein

To move from the vision to the material reality of living your dream requires some structure, a discipline to help you manifest your greatest desires, a willingness to take risks and to make mistakes.

The practice begins with *creating new beliefs and establishing clear goals* through the use of *affirmations*. Affirmations are positive statements repeated frequently, always in the present tense, containing only positive words, and serve as a response to an often-heard self-critical, limiting, or negative message, or as an expression of a need, desire, or goal.

For example, many of my chronic pain patients are very hard on themselves, and often hear their *inner critic* telling them "you should have ___" or "you could have ___ (done it differently)" or "you've made a major mistake." They might also be repeating to themselves the limiting belief they've heard from physicians, "I'll never get rid of this pain. I have to live with it."

Affirmations that would help counteract these beliefs include the following: *I love and approve of myself. I'm always doing the best I can. My (back, knee, GI tract, ___) is healthy, strong, and pain-free.* Even though the affirmations may run counter to your rational analytical mind (some people comment, "I feel like I'm lying to myself"), these positive thoughts create images that directly affect the unconscious, shaping patterns of thought to direct behavior and strongly impact desired outcomes. They act as powerful tools to unleash and stimulate the healing energy of love present in great abundance within each of us.

Keep in mind that the dismal prognosis from a physician, which might be, or feel like, a death sentence, is merely a belief. It is based on the limitations of modern medical science, a highly scientific and technologically advanced approach to the treatment of disease, and delivered to the patient by a highly educated individual in a society that defers to perceived expertise.

These negative *predictions* are quickly accepted by most patients and become a part of their own belief system. The vast majority of people with terminal diseases who accept whatever their doctors tell them (these patients are called "compliant") die very close to their predicted life expectancy. By contrast, patients who challenge their physician's "death sentence" tend to survive much longer, and some of them go on to achieve full recoveries.

Most of the beliefs held by Americans have been defined by the standards, or norms, of our parents and society, but how well does the norm fit you today, as a unique adult? If all of us attempted to conform, the world would be a boring place, devoid of creativity and innovation. We certainly wouldn't be enjoying the ease of living that technology has provided us were it not for the adventurous few who deviated from the conventional belief system.

An effective exercise for helping you become more conscious of your thoughts, beliefs, and emotions is to devote fifteen minutes *writing out all that you are thinking* during that time. Do this when you are not likely to be disturbed and don't edit anything out. After a few days of practicing this technique, many of your predominant beliefs will have been expressed on paper. Read them over. If they don't feel nurturing, build confidence and self-esteem, or regenerate and revitalize you, clearly they are not serving you and need to be either eliminated or changed.

Pay particular attention to the *shoulds*, *coulds*, and *nevers*. Before you discard what you write, examine your statements for possible clues to aspects of your life that may require more of your attention. For instance, if one of your statements reads, "I hate going to work," more than likely you may need to change your attitude about your job, or leave it for one that is more fulfilling and better suited to your talents. If the thought of leaving your job raises the thought "How will I provide for myself and my family?" then realize that this in itself can be a limiting thought. Once you liberate yourself from your old assumptions and beliefs, numerous options will become available to you, whatever they may be.

After identifying beliefs that are holding you back from your goals and desires or are negatively impacting your health, the next step is to begin to *reprogram your mind with affirmations and images* more aligned with what you want.

Most of my patients have come to me with one or more chronic physical and emotional problems. Their objectives are clear: to stop living with chronic pain, to stop having sinus infections, to eliminate their dependence on opioids, antibiotics, steroids, sleeping pills, or other medications, to have more energy, to suffer less anxiety, to get more sleep, and so forth. Once they have begun to see a definite improvement in their physical condition, which is usually after they have changed their diet and have been taking supplements for at least six to eight weeks, I recommend that they create a "wish list" in the form of affirmations.

The following is an extremely effective exercise for relieving your pain, manifesting your goals, and transforming your life.

1. List your greatest talents and gifts. You have several. These are things that are most special about you, or that you can do better than most other people. Ask yourself, "What do I most appreciate about myself?"

2. Next, list the things you most enjoy—both activities and states of being (e.g., "I love the creativity I experience with computer programming." "I really enjoy being in the mountains, or on a beach.") There will be some overlap with your first list. Many of the activities you enjoy doing are the things you're best at.

3. Next, list the things that have the most meaning for you. This is important, because if your goal doesn't meaningfully encompass more than one area of your life, or have benefit to others in some way, more than likely it is incomplete, and you will lack the passion necessary to commit to it. As you list the meaningful things in your life, you will more easily recognize the talents and activities you enjoy that are most worth your while.

4. Now make a wish list of all your goals or objectives in every realm of your life—physical, environmental, mental, emotional, social, and spiritual. Physical goals can include relieving your pain or curing your chronic condition, engaging in or mastering a challenging physical activity (e.g., running a marathon, climbing a mountain, or anything you've ever considered doing). Environmental goals might mean living

or working in a certain place. Mental goals could address career plans, financial objectives, and any limiting beliefs that you'd like to change. Emotional goals have to do with feelings and self-esteem (e.g., "I'd like to be able to identify, express, feel, or accept all of my emotions"). Social goals are about your relationships with other people (e.g., "I want more intimacy in my marriage." "I'd like to have more close friends." Or "I'd like to heal my relationship with _____ [a close friend or relative]."). Spiritual objectives have to do with your relationship with God or Spirit.

As you do this part of the exercise, ask yourself, "What does my ideal life look like?" "Where do I see myself three, five, or ten years from now?" "What is my purpose—what am I here to do?" Do *not* give yourself a time frame within which to attain any of these goals, and remember, it is *not* necessary to have a definite plan for attaining them.

5. Next, reword all of your goals into affirmations. For example, a goal might be "I'd like to be free of back pain." Some simple affirmations might be: *My back is now completely healed* or *My back feels a little better every day.* Then reduce your list to approximately ten affirmations that address your most important goals and desires (those that you'd like to have happen by tomorrow), and the most limiting beliefs or critical messages that you'd like to change. If you suffer from back pain, you may have read in Chapter 7 that back pain is often triggered by a lack of support. Effective affirmations for backache might include: *I am loved and supported. All of my needs are being met.*

After reading the section "The Issues in Your Tissues" in the chapter(s) of Part II that relate to your specific problem(s), you should be able to create at least one affirmation associated with your particular chronic pain condition.

6. Recite your entire list of affirmations at least once a day, and whenever you hear a negative, limiting, or critical message, recite the affirmation corresponding to that message. Or you can record them and listen to them in your own voice (several patients listen while in bed, as they're going to sleep). Perhaps the most effective method for deriving benefit from affirmations is to *write, recite*, then close your eyes and *visualize* them. Using this method, you would write your affirmation (have a

notebook solely for this purpose) while reciting it aloud, and then close your eyes and imagine what the affirmation looks and/or feels like, engaging as many of your senses as possible. If you can't picture them, it helps to *feel* your affirmations as you recite or write them, since this brings more energy to the experience. Make the process as vivid as possible.

I've seen several patients who have practiced this exercise daily and after sixty consecutive days reported that approximately half of their affirmations had become reality, including the resolution of severe headaches, curing of chronic sinusitis, and major improvement with several chronic pain conditions.

I worked with one woman from Tennessee via phone consultations for chronic fatigue, allergies, and sinusitis. An RN in her fifties, she taught in a nursing school in a small town and had never married, although she wanted to. She had resisted putting marriage on her goal list because, as she explained to me, "I know all the eligible men in town and in my church, and there aren't any possible candidates." I encouraged her to include it, and her affirmation read simply: *I am happily married.* Within a few months, she received a letter from a former professor with whom she'd had a friendship years earlier. His wife had died the year before, and he wanted to visit his former student. Within months they were engaged, and a year after beginning her affirmation the woman was happily married. Her tears of joy over the phone and her gratitude left me in tears as well. We both felt as if we had experienced a miracle.

The goal/affirmation or *wish list* is a dynamic process that you will continually be refining as you gain greater clarity about your needs and desires. Remember that cannabis, when used occasionally (preferably on the Sabbath) with this intention, can assist in both creating and fine-tuning your objectives and affirmations with greater specificity. It can help you to identify and trust your desires, including the possibility of *freeing yourself from the restraints of disabling chronic pain.*

LOVE YOUR BODY

The person who says it cannot be done should not interrupt the person doing it.

—Chinese proverb

An essential aspect for meeting the objective of becoming pain-free is to commit to doing whatever you possibly can to care for your body, since this is something over which you have direct control. Your next step is to begin thinking of *your body as a holy temple*, and of yourself as its caretaker. It is your most valuable possession. You are solely responsible for maintaining your body in as pristine a state as possible and for overseeing its operation at peak efficiency. Sounds like a big job, but it's actually quite simple if you focus on a few basic healthy habits.

In Part II, you've already learned how to modify your *diet* to care for your specific condition, and for most people that's the most challenging aspect of their new job. If you adhere closely to the recommended diet along with the supplements, you will most likely lose weight while also reducing pain and inflammation. Maintaining your ideal weight is important for optimal health.

I'm assuming that if you've begun implementing the MMJ and holistic medicine recommendations in Part II, you're beginning to see some progress with pain relief. By adhering to this regimen you have taken the first and most critical step in *loving your body*. I've consistently found that when your body feels fit, strong, energetic, and pain-free, you also feel healthier mentally and emotionally.

Norm Shealy, MD, PhD, and founding president of the American Holistic Medical Association, is currently eighty-four years old. He has been an inspiration and a mentor to me for nearly thirty years. In *Life Beyond 100*, he affirms that science has made it possible for humans to live until they are 140 years of age, and with good quality! That is his expectation for himself and he continues to teach others the healthy habits that will help them achieve the same result.

Now that you're on the road to recovery, you are ready for the next step in rejuvenating your body and preventing any recurrence of chronic pain. Dr. Shealy has identified four of the most basic health habits that are necessary for optimal physical well-being. For the past forty years, he has questioned his patients, students, and the public, and determined that *97 percent do not have all of the four habits* (the comments within the parentheses below are Dr. Shealy's):

- Body mass index (BMI) of 18 to 24. (Only one-third of people have this one.) To calculate yours, visit http://www.nhlbi.nih.gov/health/educational/lose_wt/BMI/bmicalc.htm.
- No smoking. (About 74 percent have this one.)
- Eat five servings of fruits and/or vegetables daily. (Only about 25 percent have this one.) One serving is equal to 2.8 ounces, but since most of us do not have a scale on our kitchen counter, I suggest you Google "one serving of fruits and vegetables." You'll be able to see what one serving looks like.
- Exercise a *minimum* of thirty minutes five days a week. (Only 10 percent of people!!)

Dr. Shealy goes on to say, "And these are only the tip of a *Titanic* of health requirements, such as adequate sleep (7 hours minimum), positive attitude, a good social network, a spiritual foundation for life, etc." I agree, but for now let's stay with his basic four and add *adequate sleep* as a fifth. Without good quality sleep it is unlikely you will be able to implement the other four. I believe it is the foundation of optimal health. If sleep has been a problem, refer to the "Insomnia" section in Chapter 15.

By complying with these five basic healthy habits, you are essentially *loving your body*. As I have repeated throughout the book, *love* is life's most powerful healer, and if you commit to these habits, you are also more likely to enjoy *loving relationships*. This aspect of life surpasses in importance all of these five basic healthy habits.

The most recent study reinforcing the healing power of love was published in April 2017. One of the longest (seventy-five years) longitudinal studies ever conducted, Harvard's Grant and Glueck study tracked the physical and emotional well-being of two populations: 456 poor men in Boston from 1939–2015 (the Grant study) and 268 male graduates from Harvard's classes of 1939–1944 (the Glueck study).

Since before World War II, they've diligently analyzed blood samples, conducted brain scans (once they became available), and pored over self-reported surveys, as well as actual interactions with these men, to compile the findings.

The conclusion? According to Robert Waldinger, director of the Harvard Study of Adult Development, "The clearest message that we get from this seventy-five-year study is this: Good relationships keep us happier and healthier. Period."

Your heart's greatest desires are your mind's way of marking the life path that will lead you to your purpose, and to feeling more fully alive. Commit now to manifesting the life of your dreams!

Conclusion
Everything in Moderation

The ultimate metaphysical secret is that there are no boundaries in the Universe.

　　　　—Ken Wilbur, an American writer on transpersonal
　　　　psychology and his own Integral Theory (1949–)

Be not afraid of changing slowly; be afraid only of standing still.

　　　　—Chinese proverb

I'm aware that some of you had already been using cannabis on a daily basis prior to reading this book . . . and for good reason. It may have been the only thing that relieved your pain, while allowing some semblance of a normal life.

　　I'm hoping that Parts II and III have helped you to significantly reduce your pain without the need for the daily use of cannabis. It's true that as a medicine, there are very few drugs as safe and effective for relieving pain as marijuana. However, if it is no longer necessary for treating your discomfort or dis-ease, then I recommend you *gradually reduce your intake to once or twice a week*, and use it primarily with a specific intention in mind. Why? Because when it is not used for treating pain and becomes a daily habit, like drinking coffee or alcohol it can lead to psychological dependence and tolerance (you may need an increasingly higher dose to obtain the desired effect). In addition it might also diminish your energy and have an adverse impact on your personality, possibly increasing anxiety, irritability, compulsivity, depression, or memory loss.

If your daily habit continues, then you'll *need* it for other than medicinal purposes, and it will lose much of its capacity to serve as your heart's compass for guiding you on your soul's path. In our current chaotic world, I consider this guidance to be one of the most beneficial qualities of cannabis, one that I've been experiencing for more than fifty years.

If you are unable to reduce your usage, then please try to consume cannabis as responsibly and safely as possible. This entails not smoking or dabbing, and carefully avoiding marijuana that is contaminated with pesticides, bacteria, fungi, or solvents. In other words, use only MMJ that is organically grown, has undergone microbial testing, and has used CO_2 in the extraction process, and if you prefer inhalation, then use a vaporizer.

There are currently twenty-eight states plus Washington, DC, that have legalized medical marijuana, comprising well over half of the U.S. population. While this medicine looks like it is here to stay, the science of cannabis is still in its infancy. However, every published study on the subject, including a January 2017 report from the National Academies of Sciences, Engineering, and Medicine entitled *The Health Effects of Cannabis and Cannabinoids: The Current State of Evidence and Recommendations for Research*, has concluded that "cannabis and cannabinoids are effective for treating pain in adults." The report also accurately states that there are *no accepted standards for the safe and appropriate use of cannabis.*

In this book, based on my professional and personal experience combined with the available scientific research, I've presented what I believe are safe and appropriate standards for using cannabis as both a medicinal and a sacred herb. This does not exclude its occasional recreational use; but too much of a good thing can become a problem. Be aware that a strong dose of self-discipline might be required to adhere to the recommendations of reduced use, and that *disciplining oneself is a critical ingredient of self-love and the key to self-healing.*

Your ultimate goal with the purchase of *Cannabis for Chronic Pain* was to free yourself from the plague of chronic pain. The book provides you with a detailed action plan and guide for achieving your objective. Maintaining an unwavering *commitment* to eliminating your pain and focusing on taking one small step at a time will greatly increase your effectiveness. Make each step its own goal, and you will feel motivated and confident about taking another step and then another.

I'm hoping that this book helps you to heal on all levels—body, mind, and spirit. Cannabis can serve you as a powerful facilitator and guide in the process of relieving your pain, transforming your life, and becoming fully alive. And the good news is that there is still so much yet to learn about the therapeutic properties of this remarkable healing herb. But what we do know is that as with any substance or activity, whether it is food, alcohol, caffeine, work, exercise, sex, or play, excessive use on a consistent basis can be harmful; and marijuana is no exception.

This book is your introduction to the self-care practice of holistic, heart-centered medicine, or *fully alive medicine*. It is a unique holistic healing manual featuring cannabis as a heart-healer of the highest order, and the primary component for quickly and safely relieving your pain.

Treat marijuana with respect and *use it sparingly but regularly as a sacred medicine*. If it is your intention, then cannabis can help you recognize the multiple causes of your pain, especially the emotional and spiritual factors and the ways in which you've deprived yourself of love; gain greater clarity on what you most need and desire and heighten the expectancy that you'll receive it; believe that *anything is possible*; trust that the feedback from marijuana is transmitted directly from your heart; become more patient, persistent, and playful; let go of the past and practice self-forgiveness; stop worrying about the future and stay focused on the present moment; become empowered, grateful, healthy, happy, and high on life! Remember, *you're always doing the best you can; there are no mistakes, only lessons;* and *everything in moderation, including moderation!*

Acknowledgments

This book serves as an introduction to the holistic subspecialty of *cannabis medicine* and my practice of *FullyAliveMedicine*. It is also a synthesis and update of various components of my ten previous books, all of which presented the specialty of *integrative holistic medicine* (IHM) and its self-care application for treating our most common chronic ailments (many of which are included in *Cannabis for Chronic Pain*), and for creating optimal health. IHM is rapidly becoming the foundation for twenty-first-century health care.

I am most grateful to my holistic physician colleagues for their commitment to pioneering this new medical specialty, and for embracing our core belief: *Love heals!* Without the mentoring and unwavering support of **Bob Anderson, MD,** my friend, fellow family physician, and cofounder of the American Board of Integrative Holistic Medicine (ABIHM), this specialty and most of my books would not exist. Bob and I worked closely together from 1993 to 2006, developing the evidence-based curriculum, creating the certification exam and the Annual 5-Day Board Review Course, and teaching and certifying physicians in IHM. There are currently more than three thousand ABIHM-certified MDs and DOs in the U.S., the majority of whom are primary care physicians. We also coauthored *The Complete Self-Care Guide to Holistic Medicine* (1999, Tarcher/Penguin). Several of the chronic pain conditions presented in *Cannabis for Chronic Pain* are updated versions of Bob's original work in the *Self-Care Guide*. Thank you, Bob, for your enormous contribution to the practice of *good medicine*, and for setting a new standard for quality health care.

In addition to Bob, who was also a cofounder and past president of the American Holistic Medical Association (AHMA), I have been mentored and inspired by several of the other cofounders of the AHMA: **Norm Shealy, MD**, founding president of AHMA; **Gladys McGarey, MD**, a past president of AHMA whose parents were both DOs who trained with Andrew Taylor. Still, MD and DO, the founder of osteopathic medicine, thus providing a strong link between osteopathy and IHM; the late **Evarts Loomis, MD**, who founded Meadowlark, the first holistic medicine retreat center in the U.S. (Hemet, California) in 1957 and the inspiration for the Fully Alive retreats; **Bernie Siegel, MD**, whose bestselling book *Love, Medicine & Miracles* provided the catalyst for my joining the AHMA in 1988, while he was serving as copresident with **Christiane Northrup, MD**, whose passion for holistic medicine was infectious; the late **Elisabeth Kübler-Ross, MD**, who in 1984, as medicine's leading authority on the subject of death and dying, radically changed my perspective on life (and death) with her article, "Death Does Not Exist"; and especially **Lev Linkner, MD**, who for nearly thirty years has been my model for the quintessential holistic family doctor, provided strong support while serving with me on the board of directors of both the AHMA and the ABIHM for more than twenty years, and has been a good friend as well.

Todd Nelson, ND, has been a significant contributor to nearly all of my ten books, as well as the coauthor of *Asthma Survival, Arthritis Survival*, and *Headache Survival*. In *Cannabis for Chronic Pain*, Todd has added his expertise to the "Holistic Medical Treatment" sections of Chapters 5, 6, 8, 9, 10, 12, and 15.

I have been working and collaborating with Todd for nearly three decades, and consider him to be among the finest holistic health practitioners in America. He is also an excellent teacher and has helped considerably with my holistic medical education. He was on the faculty of the ABIHM Annual Board Review Course for three years and was consistently among our highest-rated speakers.

Todd's practice, Tree of Life Wellness Center (www.tolwellness.com), is located in Lakewood, Colorado. There he serves patients with the most debilitating chronic conditions, the majority of whom have not responded to conventional medical treatment.

Deborah Breakell, FNP, specializes in women's health and currently practices at Helios Integrated Medicine in Boulder, Colorado, which is where we met two years ago. I've been impressed with her expertise in women's holistic health care, as evidenced by her major contribution to the "Holistic Medical Treatment" section for Dysmenorrhea in Chapter 13.

Deborah is a nationally certified family nurse practitioner through the American Nurses Credentialing Center (ANCC), with clinical experience in women's health, pediatrics, intensive care, and family practice. She is a contributing author of the book *Better Breast Health—for Life!* and shares clinical insight into women's health on www.wellcast.org. Deborah's personalized approach helps her patients achieve their health goals, using both integrative and conventional therapies.

Deborah has delivered educational presentations on the risks and benefits of hormone replacement therapy, the use of bio-identical hormones, integrative treatment options for dysmenorrhea, and other women's health issues.

Jeremy Dubin, DO, is a family physician who is also board-certified in integrative holistic medicine and addiction medicine, which is his passion. His contribution to this book is the response to Chapter 3's question 2, *Is marijuana addictive?*

Jeremy is the author of the book *The User's Guide to Not Using: An Expert Guide to Recovery from Addiction* and is a frequent speaker on the subject of addiction medicine at medical conferences nationwide and internationally. He is an assistant clinical professor in the Department of Family Medicine at the University of Colorado School of Medicine and was recently invited to teach family medicine to physicians in China.

He is also medical director of Healing Arts Recovery and Treatment Services—HEARTS, which is located in Loveland, Colorado, and his website is www.yourecovery.com.

I would also like to acknowledge **David Threlfall**, owner of two dispensaries—Trill Alternatives (Boulder) and Trill Evolutions (Denver)—

and **Lizzy Bratton,** the patient consulting manager at Trill. David has helped considerably with my training in medical marijuana as he continues to establish the industry standard for MMJ dispensaries. In addition to consistently offering a wide variety of the highest quality medical marijuana products, he and his employees provide MMJ patients with comprehensive education for using this medicine safely and effectively to treat their specific condition, based on the recorded feedback they obtain from their clientele. I know of no other dispensary tracking this data. The professionalism David has displayed, through his diligence and dedication to helping others, qualifies him as a true health care provider.

With the knowledge gained from the feedback Trill has obtained from several thousand MMJ patients/customers, Lizzy has reviewed for accuracy the MMJ recommendations in each of the chapters in Part II. I am most grateful to both David and Lizzy.

Matteo Pistono is a writer and teacher who helped immensely with the writing of the book proposal and with the editing and fine-tuning of Chapter 1.

I'm grateful to my editor, **Matthew Benjamin,** for his meticulous editing and his vision of the readership for this material. His perspective has helped considerably in shaping the book. He's done an excellent job and it's been a pleasure working with him.

Gabriel Cousens, MD, an extraordinary healer and rabbi, founder of the Tree of Life Rejuvenation Center in Patagonia, Arizona, has been one of my spiritual teachers for the past twenty years. From "Recovering the Shamanic in Judaism," Essene priest training, conscious eating, and live foods, he helped me establish much more solid footing as a physician healer. I'm also grateful to him for surprising me with a new first name, which has helped guide me through the transformation from Rob to Rav (Hebrew = spiritual teacher).

Myron McClellan served as my spiritual psychotherapist in 1986. His guidance helped cure my chronic sinusitis, and his encouragement led to my career as a health writer by inspiring *Sinus Survival*. He intuitively recognized my potential as an author (in spite of the fact I'd never written anything of consequence), ability as a healer, and opportunity to help many others suffering with chronic conditions. Myron instilled in me the healing power of love, forgiveness, intention, affirmations, and visualization; and he has continued to have a major impact on changing the course of my life. I am eternally grateful.

Lawrence Phillips, a Feldenkrais Practitioner®, has helped me become far more conscious in body, mind, and soul—in short, more *fully alive.* As a spiritual teacher along with his partner, Myron, they have been teaching *Mystical Musings* for the past fourteen years. The wisdom they share at these monthly gatherings in Denver has been an inspiration to many in our community. Through Lawrence I've learned to use cannabis more effectively as an emotional healer and as a sacred herb. And his time-management suggestions allowed me to complete the manuscript for this book on time. Thank you, Lawrence!

From **Doug Shapiro** I learned the lesson, as he exemplified the belief, that *anything's possible.* I followed his career for nearly seven of his nine active years while serving for part of that time as his personal physician/health coach as he raced throughout the United States and Europe, attempting to become the world's best cyclist. He came close, as a member of two U.S. Olympic cycling teams (1980 and 1984), as one of the first Americans to race in and complete the Tour de France, and the winner of the 1984 Coors Classic, at the time the premier American bike race. As I guided him in treating his sinus disease, he became my teacher, guinea pig, and cocreator of the Sinus Survival Program, as he continually assaulted his mucous membrane with almost daily 100-plus-mile bike rides. As a result we both were able to cure chronic sinusitis. The lessons I learned from Doug inspired me to fulfill my greatest potential as a healer and teacher and provided me with many of the necessary tools for teaching holistic medicine, treating and curing a variety of chronic conditions, achieving most of my goals, and for living with the pain of and ultimately healing shingles. Through our healing journey together, Doug has become my soul brother. Words cannot adequately express the depth of my gratitude.

Thanks to my wife, **Harriet,** for initially suggesting the idea for the book, while I was suffering through my fourth month of shingles; and for providing me with the space and incredible support to essentially work two jobs for the past year and a half, with very little playtime.

Most of all, I would like to thank my astute literary agent, **Gail Ross,** who for the past twenty-six years has provided me with a second career as an author. Gail's initial enthusiasm for *Cannabis for Chronic Pain* helped fuel my passion for this book and kept me on-task for nearly two years before publication. Her vast experience within the publishing industry and her acute awareness of what the public needs, combined with her strong commitment to making a meaningful difference, have proven to be a winning formula and brought her much deserved success. Thank you, Gail!

Resources

To receive periodic updates and current information about treating your specific chronic pain condition with the most effective MMJ products and dietary and supplement recommendations, either fax (303-447-2744) or email (info@fullyalivemedicine.com) your *Symptom Chart* and *MMJ Log* to Fully Alive Medicine, specifying your condition, email address, age, name (optional), and any comments. If you have a *success story* with MMJ that you'd like to share, please send that as well. Your feedback will contribute toward improving the quality of health care for treating and preventing chronic pain.

To find a *holistic physician* in your area certified by the American Board of Integrative Holistic Medicine go to www.abihm.org and click on "Find an ABIHM Certified Physician."

To find a *Healing Touch practitioner* certified by Healing Touch Program go to www.healingtouchprogram.com and click on "Find a Practitioner."

For the *Fully Alive Vaporizer* and *Fully Alive Alive Grinder*—go to www.fullyalivemedicine.com and click on "Fully Alive Store."

The following four cannabis products are effective for relieving pain and are available in multiple states:

- **MED-a-mints** are sublingual (under the tongue) cannabis-infused mints that provide a convenient, discreet, and healthier alternative to smoking marijuana. They effectively deliver a precise, consistent, and potent dose that lasts for four to six hours. MED-a-mints are sweetened with *xylitol*, the only sweetener recommended by the American Dental Association, with a low-glycemic index. Specific blends of pure herbs and spices are added that work synergistically with cannabis strains to either energize or relax. The three types of MED-a-mints currently available are Energizing Vanilla Mint (sativa), Exotic Chai Mint (hybrid), and Relaxing Vanilla Mint (indica). High-CBD MED-a-mints are expected soon.

Visit its website www.medamints.com for states and locations where its products can be purchased.

- **MarQaha** has created whole-plant extracted products since 2010 and specializes in creating different ingestible forms (including tinctures, edibles, and beverages) of the plant that expand your potential by offering different ways of interaction.

    Although I've been very pleased with all of their products, the 1:1/CBD:THC tincture made from Harlequin is an exceptional pain reliever. To learn more about MarQaha products visit www.marqaha.com/products.

- **LucidMood** is one of the first cannabis companies to create unique cannabinoid and terpene profiles to create specific effects. It sources individual terpenes from natural botanicals and uses CO_2 to extract all cannabinoids. There are no other additives. All LucidMood products, called "sippers," are cannabis oils that are vaporized. They each have a 1:1 ratio of CBD:THC, in addition to proprietary terpene blends that are added to create consistent and distinct effects. The current LucidMood products include four distinct moods: Bliss, Relax, Energy, and Focus; and three additional formulations: Relief, Sleep, and Cramps. Relief is an excellent choice for chronic pain, both Bliss and Relax are accurately labeled, and Focus helped me during the final ten days of editing this book.

    To find where LucidMood is sold near you, visit www.LucidMood.net.

- **CBD (Cannabidiol)**—BioCBD Plus™ is an all-natural, whole-plant, water-soluble source of CBD plus Ayurvedic herbs. What makes BioCBD unique is new technology making the product five to ten times more bioavailable in the body than traditional CBD hemp oil. These products are pesticide-free, gluten-free, and non-GMO, and contain no soy, nuts, sugar, artificial coloring, or flavoring.

    You can purchase BioCBD Plus by going to http://bit.ly/productsbiorav. The website *www.medicalsecrets.com* shares information for holistic treatments for chronic pain and other conditions with cannabis, CBD, and other natural remedies. Guided by the expert professionals in the health care industry, members of the Medical Secrets community, readers enjoy personalized service and access to the highest quality cannabis and CBD products and holistic treatments at exclusive rates.

To obtain any of the *Metagenics* supplements recommended in Part II, go to www.cfcp.metagenics.com. You can order online and the products will be shipped directly to your home. There is a 20 percent discount on your first order, and free shipping for orders over $50.00. There is also a 10 percent discount for monthly autoship plans.

To order any *Xymogen* products, go to www.xymogen.com and register using the professional code CFCP. Xymogen offers free shipping for orders that are more than $50.

To obtain *Butterbur Extra* for prevention of migraine headaches (described in Chapter 8), you can order online at www.fullyalivemedicine.com and click on Fully Alive Store.

In Chapter 3, the products mentioned for preventing increased inflammation of the respiratory mucous membrane and worsening of sinus and lung problems can be obtained by going to: https://tinyurl.com/ssccp. With the use of a onetime code, *ssccp*, you will receive free shipping with your first purchase. This procedure also applies to obtaining the candida-treatment supplements recommended in Chapter 5.

The *Sinus Survival* products include:

- Sinus Survival Herbal Nasal Spray
- Sinus Essentials Oil (peppermint + jojoba oil)
- Sinus Survival Eucalyptus Oil
- Sinus Survival Peppermint oil (for steam therapy)
- Sinus Survival Tea Tree oil (for steam therapy)
- SinuPulse Irrigation System

The *candida-treatment* supplements include:

- Allimed
- Candisol
- Candicide
- LateroFlora
- Sinus Survival Pro Biotic

For ten- to twenty-eight-day *Functional Medicine Detoxification Programs and Gut Restoration* programs, contact Todd Nelson, Naturopath, at 303-969-3052, or www.tolwellness.com to schedule in-office, telephone, or Skype visits.

Functional Medicine Lab Testing—In several chapters I recommend functional medicine lab testing. When seeking holistic care, make sure the practitioner uses one of the following labs to determine underlying imbalances and causes of your chronic pain.

- Genova Diagnostics: www.gdx.net
- Cyrex Laboratories: www.cyrexlabs.com

- Pharmsan Labs: www.pharmasan.com
- Diagnos-Techs: www.diagnostechs.com

There are multiple sites on the Internet to learn more about the most recent **cannabis research**, including: www.webmd.com, http://www.cmcr.ucsd .edu/, and https://nccih.nih.gov/health/marijuana.

The Scientist on YouTube (www.youtube.com/watch?v=csbJnBKqwIw) is a documentary of Dr. Mechoulam, discoverer of THC and "father of cannabis science."

Medical Secrets (www.medicalsecrets.com) shares information for holistic treatments for chronic pain and other conditions with cannabis, CBD, and other natural remedies. Guided by the expert professionals in the health care industry, members of the Medical Secrets community enjoy personalized service and access to the highest quality cannabis and CBD products and holistic treatments at exclusive rates.

For contemporary *spiritual teaching* from Myron McClellan and Lawrence Phillips and their *Mystical Musings*, go to mysticalmusings.net to learn more about its monthly Musing and to sign up for its mailing list. You can also download Mystical Musings Podcasts for free by going to iTunes, click on the iTunes Store, and search for Mystical Musings.

To learn more about *holistic self-care*, visit www.fullyalivemedicine.com and click on:

- "Fully Alive Education"—Dr. Rav's blog with information about webinars, CDs, DVDs, seminars, workshops, and conferences, plus updates on recent medical marijuana research.
- "Fully Alive Retreats"—ten-day, three- and six-week residential retreats oriented towards one of the following:

  1. *Chronic Dis-ease*—focus on healing many of our most common chronic conditions, including the majority of those presented in Part II
  2. *Healing-the-Healer*—for health care practitioners
  3. *Conscious Living*—for individuals, couples and families interested in creating optimal health, thriving relationships, and functional families
  4. *Optimal Performance*—for business executives, athletes, musicians, artists— those individuals and groups interested in realizing their greatest potential while fully utilizing their talents and gifts both individually and as a group/ team

- "Fully Alive Camps"—three-week residential camp programs for children between the ages of eight and seventeen.
- "Fully Alive Medical Centers"—to find a FAM Center near you.

Index

About the Author

May my love of the art of medicine inspire me to seek at all times to expand my knowledge and to see within each of those in need, only the human being.

—Moses Maimonides, a physician and rabbi (1135–1204)

Dr. Robert (Rav) Ivker is a holistic healer, family physician, cannabis clinician, health educator, and bestselling author of ten books, most notably *Sinus Survival: The Holistic Medical Treatment for Sinusitis, Allergies, and Colds.* He is a board-certified holistic physician (ABIHM), the cofounder and past president of the American Board of Integrative Holistic Medicine, a past president of the American Holistic Medical Association (AHMA), a fellow of the American Academy of Family Physicians, and a certified Healing Touch practitioner.

Dr. Rav received his DO degree from the Philadelphia College of Osteopathic Medicine and began practicing medicine in 1972 as a family doctor. During the past six years in his Fully Alive Medicine practice in Boulder, Colorado, he has evaluated and worked with nearly seven thousand patients seeking a license issued by the Colorado Department of Public Health and Environment to legally obtain medical marijuana. Well over 90 percent of these patients were suffering with chronic pain.